As You Wish

Light In the Darkness of AIDS

As You Wish

Light in the Darkness of AIDS

By

Christine Massot Simpson

Rainbow's End Company
354 Golden Grove Road
Baden, PA 15005

Published by Rainbow's End Company
354 Golden Grove Road
Baden, PA 15005

http://adpages.com/rbebooks/light.htm
email btucker833@aol.com

Printed in the United States of America

Publisher's Cataloging-in-Publication
(Provided by Quality Books, Inc.)

Simpson, Christine Massot.
    As you wish : light in the darkness of AIDS / Christine Massot
Simpson. -- 1st ed.
    p. cm.
    Preassigned LCCN: 97-68911
    ISBN: 1-880451-25-5

    1. Simpson, Gary, 1961- --Health. 2. Simpson, Christine Massot
--Marriage. 3. AIDS (Disease)--Patients--Biography.   I. Title.

RC607.A26S55 1997   362.1'969792'0092
                         QBI97-30292

Dedicated in memory of my sister . . . Brigitte,
who now understands the big picture.

Cover Design: Susan Vincent

Cover Illustration: Gary Simpson

Contents

"Aimer, ce n'est pas se regarder l'un l'autre, mais regarder ensemble dans une même direction." Antoine de Saint Exupéry

Chapter One

Which Road?

Anxious to be back with Gary, I hurried down the bleak hospital corridor. At my sister's insistence, I had reluctantly agreed to take a much-needed break with her. Gary's room was located on the quiet, second-floor ward of this small university hospital; but, as I neared the area, I was immediately caught up in a frenzy of nurses and doctors who were wheeling my fiancé to the Intensive Care Unit. My thoughts raced, *There's an oxygen tank secured to the side of his hospital bed. This means he can't breathe properly! How could this have happened? What's wrong?*

Although I don't think I asked these questions aloud, I heard someone say, "Conditions have gotten worse. Please, can you get Gary's personal belongings and follow us to the IC Unit?" I nodded my head and, then, quickly and mechanically, gathered his possessions. My mind couldn't absorb what was happening. It was too much, too fast!

"I love you Gary," I said over and over to him as we followed the entourage of medical professionals. Holding his hand tightly, I realized that I needed to be strong for him. *Just hang on,* I said to myself. *You can't break down now.* My heart pounded loudly as I fought to control my emotions. Gary's words, though barely audible, encouraged me. "I love you," he mouthed back. Eventually I was to become very good at lip reading—especially those particular words.

Once inside Gary's sterile glass-walled room, the beep of the heart monitor and the hiss of the oxygen were unsettling. As he lay there, trying desperately to breathe with probes gelled to his chest, back and temples, I felt frightened and helpless. This was definitely not the type of visual stimulation I needed to help me be an effective encourager. *What must Gary be thinking and feeling?* His arms were sore, his entire body ached, and the oxygen was going at 100 percent. Being weak from not eating didn't help much. At that moment, with both of us feeling so very vulnerable, only prayer and reading from the Bible could settle, soothe, and comfort us.

The following passages were especially meaningful to the two of us:

Be strong and courageous. Do not be afraid or terrified . . .
for the Lord your God goes with you:
he will never leave you nor forsake you.

Deuteronomy 31:6

The Lord is my shepherd, I shall not be in want;
He makes me lie down in green pastures,
he leads me beside quiet waters,
he restores my soul.
He guides me in the path of righteousness for his name's sake.
Even though I walk through the valley of the shadow of death,
I will fear no evil, for you are with me;

your rod and your staff; they comfort me.
You prepare a table before me in the presence of my enemies.
You anoint my head with oil;
my cup overflows.
Surely goodness and love will follow me all the days of my life,
and I will dwell in the house of the Lord forever.

Psalm 23

For my thoughts are not your thoughts
neither are your ways my ways . . .
As the heavens are higher than the earth,
so are my ways higher than your ways
and my thoughts than your thoughts.

Isaiah 55:8-9

"I can do everything through Him who gives me strength."

Philippians 4:13

Chapter Two

The Diagnosis

There were no immediate answers to what was wrong with Gary. Though he fought with much determination and will, he was obviously suffering great physical and emotional pain. Frustrated with trying to talk, he would point to the things he needed. After simply brushing his teeth, his pulse rate would escalate to 120 beats per minute. It hurt immeasurably to see this young man, who meant so much to me, enduring such pain; however, I was determined to be a source of strength for him. Staying by his side over the next few days, I prayed that he could sense and feel my hope for our future. *God had a plan, but what was it?*

A nurse, concerned because I wasn't getting enough sleep, and knowing I wouldn't go home, gave me an alternative. "You can use the adjoining room, if you like," she offered. "But, please, please, get some rest. You're absolutely exhausted."

Finally, I agreed. "It will help just knowing that Gary is close by. But, I can't—I just can't leave."

"I understand," she said and, somehow, I knew that she did.

When I awoke on Sunday morning, I thought, *What better way to be greeted than by a loving wave from one's best friend, even through glassed walls, from one hospital bed to another.* We had enough uncertainties in our lives without being separated. Biopsies had revealed nothing that could put a name to his illness. In the meantime, we tried to strengthen Gary with protein mixes, milkshakes, juices, barley greens, soups . . . anything absorbable through a straw.

God, I thought, *please give the doctors an answer. No more guessing games. It happened quickly, so please end it quickly.* Instantly, this last thought retraced its path through my mind.

Had it really happened so quickly? I went back to a time several months earlier . . .

In June, Gary had qualified to swim at the Paralympics—the Olympic Games for the physically disabled in Seoul, Korea that fall. Then the month of August took him to a training camp in Holland with many Canadian amputee swimmers. Although Gary had lost a leg in his early years, he hadn't allowed this to interfere with his living a full life, and meeting special challenges. It was difficult for me to even remember that he was an amputee—it was just a word to describe a condition—not him. The training camp was a mixture of social activities, hard work, and, unfortunately, sickness. The damp quarters and daily training resulted in fatigue and illness, which led to the entire team returning from Holland feeling poorly. Although some were able to shake off their illness, others saw doctors and were prescribed medication against this Dutch bug. Gary, however, for some reason, was hesitant to have things checked out.

When I visited him daily at his basement suite, a stone's

throw away from my housing accomodation on Vancouver's west side, I would prod and coax him to see the team doctor. But he was evasive and would not agree. "I think," he finally said, "that I'd like to find a Christian physician." I tried to let it go but as he battled fevers, night sweats, and nausea while trying to make it through his day as a special education teacher in Abbostsford, a forty-five minute commute from Vancouver, I became frightened and confused. *Why doesn't he go to the doctor?* I wondered. *Is there something he's afraid to talk about?* Gary, feeling more and more fatigued, prayed with me that he would find a good physician—someone he could trust. Through referrals he did find a new GP very close to home who, in turn, led him to another doctor. This professional was a specialist at UBC.

The word specialist did not reassure me. *Was Gary really that sick? Was his condition that serious?* My mind began going over what I considered to be possibilities? I even thought about the worse-case scenario—that of Gary having AIDS. Before our engagement, he had shared with me about past mistakes—things he had done that he was sorry for, ashamed of, and concerned about. He had also seemed somewhat frightened; however, both of us chose not to dwell on the past, knowing how damaging that can be. I didn't want to know the details.

I tried to erase the word AIDS from my mind. *No! It can't be,* I thought. Though I had somewhat come to terms in admitting that there was the *possibility* of a sexual relationship—perhaps a homosexual one—having caused his illness, I refused to accept the diagnosis of a fatal disease. *I loved the Gary that I now knew, the Gary who had become a new person in Christ. We'd gone through so many trials in our relationship, and we'd get through this one, too.* The new-found doctor was an answer to prayer—a treasure. He not only treated his patients as individuals but believed in the power of God. He prayed with us, asking that God be with us every step of our journey. Both Gary and I trusted him, and, moreover, we trusted God to see us through this.

It was Gary who gave me the diagnosis after getting the report. His drawn face told me that it was serious. "I've got— I've got AIDS." It was difficult to understand him—difficult for the choking words to penetrate his heart-breaking, broken sobs. "I'm so sorry, Christine. So very sorry. I love you so much."

Although devastated and torn apart by his words, I tried to appear strong, choosing my words carefully. "We'll see this through together. I love you; we love one another. Somehow, we'll make it work." Inwardly, I rebelled at this bombshell. All I knew about AIDS and HIV was that it was a virus—one other people got. Not someone I knew, let alone someone I was going to marry!

I lift up my eyes to the hills-
where does my help come from?
My help comes from the Lord,
the Maker of heaven and earth.

Psalm 121:1-2

"Dear friends, do not be surprised at the painful trial you are suffering . . . But rejoice that you participate in the sufferings of Christ, so that you may be overjoyed when His Glory is revealed."

1 Peter 4:12-13

Chapter Three

How Do We Tell Them?

Gary had been suffering from pneumocystis carinii, a lung infection that causes severe shortness of breath and a heavy cough. Most persons are subjected to this form of pneumonia only during childhood, but because of Gary's immune deficiency, he developed the infection.

We were in a life and death situation and our families had to be told. *But what was the best way to handle it?* After things settled down in the ICU, I called my mother and father. "Maman, Papa, the doctors know what's wrong with Gary. We're in ICU." My short choppy sentences sounded strange even to myself. "He has pneumonia and . . . and he has AIDS." In response to their shock and words of concern and love, I began to sob. My mind issued a silent plea. *Please, tell me that it's going to be all right. Tell me!* But, of course, they couldn't. No one could.

The doctor made calls to Gary's mother, who in turn was to contact his father in Havelock, Ontario, a brother in Calgary, and other family members in the Lower Mainland of Vancouver. Realizing that his young patient was in a life-threatening situation, he wanted the family present. When I told Gary that his father was coming to see him, he was very upset. "Why? Why is he coming?" he asked.

"Out of love and concern and wanting to see for himself that everything is going to be all right," I said, trying to reassure him. Perhaps the reality of the situation had not quite sunk in for me, but I truly believed that Gary was going to pull through. After all, just a month earlier, we had announced our engagement. *Such celebration,* I thought. *Such joy, excitement, and love. Had it been shattered? Dare I have hope for a future?*

I was teaching a seventh grade French Immersion Class in a nearby school district at the time and, the following Monday, it was necessary for me to return to the classroom. Although in a daze, I somehow performed my teaching duties. Priorities began to shift and efficient time management became an art. Socializing outside of class with colleagues was non-existent, and my breaks were spent checking in on Gary by telephone or making plans for the following day.

Although my colleagues knew that my fiancé was in the hospital, no one was fully aware of the gravity of the situation. Nor was I prepared right then to tell them.

My daily routine was the same. After leaving school promptly at 3:00 p.m., with everything in order for the next day, I returned to the sterile solemnity of the Intensive Care Unit.

With a tear-streaked face that inevitably happened during the forty minute drive, I'd approach the front desk hesitantly. "Is . . . is it okay to go in?"

The nurses always spoke with compassion. "Yes, of

course, maybe you can do something." This one time, Gary was at an all-time emotional low, heartbroken and devastated, believing that our hope for the future had been destroyed by the diagnosis of AIDS.

"Dad was in to see me . . . my brother, too. I told them and others as well. I . . . I can't take this, Christine." Each acknowledgment of the disease and every reminder of the virus was like repeating his death sentence. The words reinforced and confirmed the worst in his mind. Suddenly, the unanswered questions and tension he had been living with for so long demanded an outlet for release. "Oh, Christine I don't want to leave you. I don't want to go. I want a family— my own children. Please, please, don't go away from me."

Although the doors had always been open for me to leave, I knew the Lord would grant us the strength we needed. "Gary," I vowed, "please know that we are going to make it. Never, ever, will I leave you!" Crying unashamedly, I continued, "This I promise, knowing that God wants us to be together. And, as for a family, well, we could adopt. We'll allow God to lead us in all our decisions."

Therefore I tell you, do not worry about your life . . .
Who of you by worrying can add a single hour to his life?
Since you cannot do this very little thing,
why do you worry about the rest?

Luke 12:22, 25-26

"Wait for the Lord; be strong and take heart and wait for the Lord."

Psalm 17:14

Chapter Four

Groundwork for Marriage

Following the initial diagnosis and the first treatments, I took two days off from school to see Gary out of Intensive Care and on to a strength-building road of recovery. *We are going to make it,* I told myself over and over again. *We have to!*

Both of us rejoiced when Gary was discharged from the hospital after a four-week stay. We were physically exhausted and emotionally drained from the ordeal. The gratitude we felt for being able to spend time together outside of glassed walls was indescribable. The bleak hospital routine had been washed with the jubilant colors of victory and triumph. Gary had survived the pneumonia and, as long as we were together, we could handle the AIDS issue. Over time it became clear that treatment with Pentamadine, a drug that drastically reduces blood counts, was producing positive results. In November he also began taking AZT (Zidovudine) which had been in use since 1986. It was a costly antiviral drug which reduced the level of viral replication and the spread of the infection to new cells. We were told that side effects included anemia (low red blood cell count), neutropenia (low white blood cell count), as well as muscle deterioration. I wanted to do something to help with the mental and physical strain Gary suffered from the depressing drug therapy—two pills every four hours . . . and so I bought him a special watch with five alarms for his birthday. That way, he wouldn't miss his "med" time and suffer adverse side effects. The watch was a superb help but there was also a dark side to this birthday present. Whenever his watch beeped, it also reminded us that he had a fatal disease and that, with each passing moment, some of our precious time had lapsed.

We kept reminding ourselves that God had a plan, and we were not about to give up on what He had for us. Without Him, our situation would have cast an unbearable shadow of darkness and despair upon us and our plans for the future. There would have been no hope. Of course, we couldn't ignore the toll on our lives that this disease had brought about. As Gary coped with the unpredictable side effects of fevers and extreme fatigue, we both struggled with anger and depression. But we never gave up our dreams for a future together and were looking forward to being married. *But*, we wondered, *how would others feel about us taking this step?* We anticipated disapproval and rejection from friends and, possibly, even family members.

We received much support from Gary's family in our plans to marry. "We're happy that marriage is still a part of your plans," they said reassuringly. "We know there is risk for you, and have great respect for your determination to go ahead with such a joyous celebration."

I'd never turn away from him, I thought. *Never!*

Seated in my parent's living room, tense, tearful and tired, we told my family about our plans. Their reaction was, understandably, not as supportive. They were concerned and very frightened for me. My father sounded intense, "How can you both expect to lead a normal married life without Christine contracting the disease?" Then he went on to answer his own question. "You can't! It's impossible!"

I forced my voice to sound calm as I held back my tears. "Papa, we know we will have limitations and restrictions. We're aware of all the dangers and are ready to deal with them. God will give us the strength." My mother sat on the sofa by the wall, her sobs and tears bringing momentary fear and doubt to my mind. *They're positive that we have no future*, I thought. *They are convinced that my life will be ruined.*

"It would be irresponsible." Dad's words echoed my mother's distraught look.

I could sense the tension building within Gary. The look on his face told me that he felt this was a personal attack. But, I knew it was the disease he had, not him, that they feared. They didn't want to lose me.

"Christine, it's no use," Gary said defensively. "They're not listening to us. Come on; let's go!" He got up, grabbed his shoes, and headed for the door.

Not wanting to leave things the way they were, I said, "No, Gary. We have to talk about it. Please, try to understand their concerns."

And so, once again, the four of us sat down. My father broke the silence. "We . . . we love you both. But surely you can see the dangers involved. Can't you just be best friends? At least hold off on marriage plans for awhile."

"Papa, I appreciate your fear and concern, but God will give us the strength to deal with potential obstacles. We know that we will have to make sacrifices, but we are committed in our love and trust that God will help us."

Determined to stick with the vow I had made to Gary, the man I loved, I thought, *Only God can change my mind.* We left the house with unsatisfied and uneasy feelings in our hearts. We had very much wanted their blessing. Perhaps, it would yet happen.

Gary's disease scared many people away, in spite of the increased awareness and educational efforts being made to inform people about HIV and AIDS. Many of our days, weeks, and months were filled with frustration, hurt, and feelings of rejection. Fear of the unknown runs deep. There were some people who outright showed their objections to our wedding plans. Others did not want Gary near their children for fear of chance injuries and still "unknown" causes of HIV. Gary and I both loved children and were used to demonstrating this love openly and joyfully. When hugs and playing with children was out of the question, that joy was ripped away, adding deep wounds to our already bleeding hearts. Even though I was "allowed" to be with the children, I purposely did not involve myself with them too often, trying to spare Gary from the painful reminder of what he couldn't do. Although we disagreed with peoples' fears, there was nothing we could do but respect their wishes and pray. We could not change them; however, we were called to love them.

The two of us never gave up on God and tried to capture tiny glimpses of light at the end of our tunnel. We obviously needed all the help and support that was available. I recalled a female doctor at the hospital who had given me some advice after I learned the truth about Gary's diagnosis. Pulling me aside abruptly, she advised, "You're going to need some help. You need to talk to someone." I decided she was right and, after talking with Gary, made an appointment with a counselor at the local AIDS Center for sometime in January.

When the day of the appointment finally arrived, I was somewhat apprehensive as I approached the front desk. "I . . . I have an appointment with a counselor; my name is Christine."

"Oh, yes, Christine," she replied, pointing to a room. "We'll talk there. Go on in. I'll be with you in just a moment." Two empty chairs sat at angles to one another; the

24

view from the window was grey and wet. Questions burned within me and, when she joined me, I didn't waste time. "My fiancé and I are seeking God's will in our wish to marry; however, I want to know if you are aware of any other couples who have gone through this."

She hesitated. "Well, I know of one person whose husband became ill with AIDS after marriage—"

Impatiently, I interrupted her. "But what about before marriage? Is there another woman I can talk with who had to make the same decision that I am making?"

"Unheard of! Simply unheard of!"

Convinced that our situation was unique, I never returned to the agency. Although the counselor listened with compassion, she could not easily identify with my quest for God's will in our situation.

Searching for counseling elsewhere, I was referred to the then-chaplain at St. Paul's Hospital in Vancouver. This time Gary went with me to see this Catholic priest who dealt primarily with persons with AIDS. We felt he should be a good candidate to offer us advice. Seated behind his desk, the robust man spoke. "Welcome, what can I do for the two of you?"

After some disclosure, Gary sat silently, as I talked. "We are seeking God's will in our wish to marry. We are surely not ignorant. Do you think it would be wrong for us to marry, given our limitations?"

He looked directly at both of us, obviously trying to see beyond surface appearances. "Well," he began, "people marry because they love each other and are committed. I see that you meet these conditions. However, a natural expression of this deep love is sexual intercourse, and there would obviously be limitations for you. Seeing that you do understand the implications of the disease, and are willing to use measures to prevent further spread of the disease to you, Christine, and seeing that you truly love and care for each other, let me review this situation with my superiors in Rome. I am going next week and will be sure to confer with them on this issue."

We felt satisfied with his answer, believing he had not shunned our wishes. Both Gary and I believed that there could be no "wrong" in this situation since we put God first in our lives and trusted that He would strengthen us in our marriage. In reality, I think we were just doing groundwork, so that others, primarily my parents, could, in turn, speak to reputable people who supported our heartfelt desires.

After another referral, we ventured out to Burnaby Christian Counseling Center where we were matched up with separate counselors knowledgeable about AIDS.

Both of us were told by our counselor that they knew of no similar situation, but that they believed we could work things out. It was beneficial seeing separate counselors since we were seeking God's will as individuals and as a couple. Both of us had questions. *Was this disease a sign that we weren't to marry?* We didn't think so and neither did the counselors. Encouraged by their support, we also met with a premarital counselor at the Center. The light began to flicker a little brighter. Then a couple from our church added more intensity to the flame as they, too, supported our fervent desires.

We finally set a tentative date for our wedding. Since the church we attended already had a wedding booked on that day, we made inquiries at one of my favorite Catholic churches. I knew one of the priests from my high school days —a very accepting, open-minded, and humorous man. There was no doubt in my mind that Gary would like him, but would this priest marry us? When we disclosed our story to him, his response resounded loud and clear. "So, what are we waiting for? Let's get on with it." He did not doubt our love or pass judgment. God was with us.

In the meantime, the other Catholic priest had returned

from Rome with more support. My parents, both Catholics, spoke with the priests and also with our friends from the church. They came to understand that we knew what we were dealing with, trusted God, had an authentic love for one another, and that, indeed, great things were possible. We were over one hurdle. Gary's journal entry for June 25, 1989 expresses how he felt about this:

> So much has happened!! Our prayers have been answered and, yes, in two weeks we'll be Mr. and Mrs.!!! In Feb/Mar, Christine and I attended counseling sessions to have other opinions on our situation. Priests, ministers, church people, all agreed that what we want is ok in God's eyes.

It should have been a wonderful and joyous time for the bride-to-be, but my three roommates knew that there was something bothering me. They observed that I spent countless hours in my bedroom, obviously avoiding them. Gary and I had experienced so much rejection that I wasn't ready for any more—nor did I want to cry on his shoulders all the time. After all, he was facing every day with thoughts of life and death.

Gary, feeling hurt and embarrassed, had difficulty explaining his mixed-up emotions. Once, when asked by a colleague if he had AIDS, he denied it, yet in his journal, said that he wanted to tell his friend then, but was afraid. Gary prayed for patience, love in the families, and wisdom and peace in his heart as he battled confusion and anger towards those who spoke against our marriage and future plans.

When one of my roommates heard me crying over the whole situation, she perched herself on the edge of my bed. "Christine, please tell me what is wrong!"

Giving in to the need to tell someone other than a family member, I spilled out all my feelings to her. We shared tears of pain and sadness which seemed to, momentarily, ease some of my hurt. From then on this roommate was a significant friend and help to both of us. Many people followed.

We kept silent at our respective work places, giving people vague answers about wedding plans. Disclosing our situation to certain persons would have put them in a difficult position. We didn't know how they would react to the news, and each disclosure seemed to bring on an onslaught of emotional pain for all involved. Gary and I didn't want to burden others with our problems, and neither one of us felt it was fair to tell others and then ask them not to say anything until we felt the time was right.

Through counseling, making marriage plans, and our never-ending quest for God's will in our lives, we realized that the roots that held our love steadfast dug deeper in richer faith, thus, chances of us growing apart was impossible. As our love grew daily, our priorities became more focused.

The Spirit himself testifies with our spirit that we are God's children. Now if we are God's children, then we are heirs . . . of God and co-heirs with Christ if indeed we share in his sufferings in order that we may also share in his glory.
I consider that our present sufferings are not worth comparing with the glory that will be revealed in us . . .
For in this hope we were saved. But hope that is seen is no hope at all. Who hopes for what he already has? But if we hope for what we do not yet have, we wait for it patiently.
In the same way, the spirit helps us in our weakness. We do not know what we ought to pray for, but the spirit himself intercedes for us . . .
And we know that in all things God works for the good of those who love him, who have been called according to his purpose.

Romans 8:16-18, 24-26, 28

"If life is a journey, how do you know when you've arrived?"

Chapter Five

Beginnings

Gary and I both firmly believed that we had been brought together by God and that He would give us the strength to meet the challenges of each day. Our relationship had developed rather slowly over several years; however, from the very beginning I found Gary intriguing. When we met, I had just completed my first year at the University of British Columbia and was looking forward to my life-guarding job with the Vancouver Parksboard. Maple Grove Park is nestled in the heart of a beautiful Vancouver neighborhood, shaded with sturdy old trees with strong roots . . . that apparently caused havoc to the pool each year. At the preliminary staff meeting, I studied the four new faces and wondered what it was going to be like to get to know these people. Day one's on-site action helped in these efforts. With no children around, we spread out a blanket, sat down and began to talk—our first four-hour stint became an attempt to get to know one another.

One fellow named Gary fascinated me. Although he was

a world class swimmer, he wasn't the "show off" type. I was curious and tried to initiate some conversation.

"Where's your family from?"

"Oh, all over. We moved a lot."

"Do you have any brothers or sisters?"

"Yeah, there are eight children."

"Eight!" I echoed in astonishment.

As he positioned himself comfortably on the blanket, he offered a simple explanation. "Both of my parents remarried." Then he closed his eyes, obviously ready for a nap.

It sure isn't going to be easy to get to know this guy, I thought. Talk about insight. Little did I know!

I soon learned that Gary's schedule was one of precision. When he was not out of town competing, he had swim workouts at 5:00 a.m. and also after work hours. Somewhere, in between, there might be a weight workout. I began to understand why napping was a necessity for him.

My time and energy, during the work day, was spent getting to know the "regulars" at Maple Grove Park, french braiding hair in time for local birthday parties, monitoring mothers who assumed we would babysit their non-swimming children, and, on rainy days, becoming progressively more adept at Trivial Pursuit and card games.

I enjoyed my job. All of the staff got along exceptionally well and vowed to return the following summer. Gary, it seemed, was not the quiet person that I had met the first day. He was a warm, kindhearted, energetic individual who was fun to be around. I considered him a friend, but socially, outside of work hours, we led separate lives. Although Gary's left leg had been amputated below the knee as a young child, he had begun swimming at the age of twelve with the Surrey Knights Swim Club.

"I needed to exercise to get rid of my roly-poly appearance," he said, chuckling.

"Well, it worked," I commented, surveying his 5' 9" frame,

curly brown hair, and lean, tanned body. "You look great!" His response was a wide, generous smile.

"I think if it hadn't been for the accident, I could have been a gymnast. Sometimes, I really wonder what it would be like to run across a field, or maybe run with a dog, leaving the earth far behind, beneath my feet." His stunning, light-blue eyes had a dreamy look.

Surprised by this admission, I said nothing, hoping he would go on to share some more information with me. I was genuinely interested in this man who seemed to have so much to give to others. His fun-loving ways and cheerful nature caused people to want to be around him. They could tell he was really interested in them and, even more importantly, that he believed in them. Gary worked successsfully with physically and mentally disabled persons in various settings. The more I learned about him, the more intrigued I was. Eventually, as our friendship deepened, I asked many questions about his family, his involvement in swimming, and his amputation. Slowly, through his words, and, later, through those of his mother, I was able to piece together what had happened to his leg . . .

He had been six at the time and had a new bike. It was early morning and Gary, ready to leave the house, asked his mother a question. "Can I please ride my bike to school? Please! I'll be careful."

Since Gary was capable and responsible, and his older brother would be riding along with him, his mother agreed. She had hesitated momentarily because his sister didn't have a bicycle and wouldn't be able to ride with them. Minutes later, his mother heard the sound of brakes screeching and piercing shrieks. Terrified, she feared the worst.

Gary, coming down the hill from Main Street, had failed to navigate a right turn onto Center Street, in Delta, a surburb of Vancouver. His brother, who was ahead of him, saw the truck to the left and thought that Gary would be able to slow down, turn, or stop. He couldn't and didn't! The impact of the front end of the 33-foot empty Kenworth truck left a 169 foot skid mark. Unfortunately, Gary's left leg was crushed underneath the wheels! An ambulance transported him to the hospital where a bone specialist made an on-the-spot decision to amputate his leg below the knee. He also had numerous cuts and bruises to his head, and a broken back. It was necessary for him to have a tracheotomy. Because the diagnois was so discouraging, he was baptized in the hospital. However, it was not to be the last time the medical field underestimated Gary Simpson.

Once doctors operated on his spine, Gary's courage and love of life allowed him to be wheeled out of the Intensive Care Unit. After bone was grafted from his right leg to fuse the spine, he was strapped to a Foster Bed for six weeks. Terrified, he learned to deal with the pain and confusion. He was discharged from the hospital on Christmas Day with orders to have a checkup in six weeks. This turned out fine; however, in March all were shocked to discover that his spine had not fused. There was no determination if it had come unfused or was improperly done. Hundreds of miles away from home, at a hospital in Winnipeg, Manitoba, this time using grafted bone from his hip, another attempt was made to fuse his back. This time a Foster Bed was part of his life for almost four months. He was then fitted for a plastic type cast for his back, given a prosthesis and released.

When Gary ventured off to class in September, because of constant medical problems, his parents drove him to and from school. In January of that school year, almost a year and a half since the accident, Gary's mother, saw the terrible pain he was in, and realized that he needed further evaluation. She felt something else had to be wrong! But the doctors disagreed, built up his right shoe, and sent mother and son home. Other specialists from various fields said the same thing. Months later, after a counselor had helped the young

Gary work through his emotions, the family doctor said, "the boy is trying to rule his mother."

Finally, disappointed with local doctors, the family moved to Rutland, in the interior of British Columbia. Gary was still in incredible physical pain. The local doctor in Rutland knew that indeed there was a problem. Once x-rays were taken and evaluated, it was determined that an injured right hip had not healed properly. The patient was sent to a doctor in Kelowna who, in turn, referred Gary to B. C. Children's Hospital in Vancouver where a plate and pin were inserted in his hip. Being a growing boy, the bones in his stump would pierce the healed skin over and over again, and yet another operation would have to be performed. Then he had to have the tibia bone of his stump shortened. Infections were always a risk. Finally, after a long period of teachers' visits at home, Gary started grade five at South Rutland School. His keen mind and enthusiasm for learning enabled him to keep up with his peers.

Phantom pains were part of Gary's childhood as well as his adult life. Neither the cause, nor the intractable pain that would race through his amputated leg, have been fully explained by researchers. There was evidence of the vivid reality of the multiple sensations he experienced, when he would feel his toes, wiggle them, or even get a cramp in his foot. It was as though his leg were still there. The sensation of cramps in his shin or his foot were the most excruciating. It is believed that the nerve endings severed upon amputation continue to generate impulses to the individual's brain.

Although Gary went through a lot in his early years, he grew to be a knowledgeable and successful individual who was able to get involved in swimming and, through the Canadian Amputee Sports Association, competed internationally. Many times he said, "You know Christine, the accident was the best thing that could have happened to me. It shaped me into the person I am. I had to learn to fight for my goals."

That may be true, I thought, *but God created you. If only you believed in Him. What a difference it would make.*

Ask and it will be given to you; seek and you will find; knock and the door will be opened to you.

Matthew 7:7

"Love one another deeply and from the heart"

1 Peter 1:22

Chapter Six

The Wheels of Love

Whenever I saw someone a distance away who was wearing a UBC swim team jacket, I always strained my eyes and neck to see if I recognized the one wearing it. Once, during my second year of school, that person was Gary. The pitter patter in my heart crescendoed above that of the rain. *Ok, Christine, calm down,* I said to myself, as he stopped to greet me. Automatically, I reached up to smooth my short brown hair, wishing I had spent a little more time on it that morning. *What was it about Gary that made me feel so so—?*

Before I could figure out how he made me feel, I was staring into his friendly, inquisitive, clear-blue eyes. "Christine, it's great to see you. How is life treating you?"

"Fine!" I swallowed hard. "And you, how . . . how have you been?"

"Great! Will you be working at Maple Grove this summer?"

"I'm hoping to."

"That's good. Me, too."

After a few more moments of casual conversation, we went our separate ways. My fascination with this man had led me to keep track of his many victories through the local papers.

Do I have to make the papers before he takes a real interest in me? I wondered. *Will he ever see me as more than a casual friend?*

It didn't happen during our second summer at Maple Grove. It was a time of work, good times, and laughter. There were times that Gary and I even went out as friends, and it seemed that the more time I spent with him, the more I admired and respected him as a person. He loved children and always took the time to talk with them, offering encouragement and support.

It was obvious that he would be a good father. When I mentioned this he said, "That's definitely in my future. I want to have children."

"I'm sure they'll be great swimmers if they're to be anything like their father."

Keeping tabs of his international competitions in the summer was easy. He would send postcards and then tell us all his stories when he returned. He kept travel journals, recording thoughts of people, places, and events. Everyone at Maple Grove found him interesting and was impressed by his boundless energy and cheerful disposition. All too soon the summer ended; however, I was excited that I would be spending the third year of my undergraduate study at Université Laval just outside of Quebec City.

Being on my own in this distant place made it a challenging year. Although the language was never a barrier, the long, cold winter found me lonely at times. I became adept at knitting; a group of Vancouverites (among others) would meet weekly to knit and chat. On Sundays I would venture out to church, feeling a need to be with God. Although I knew that God was always with me, I felt the desire to be in a place that honored Him. In the middle of a service, I would often find myself in tears. "Oh, Lord," I would pray. "Give me some direction. Fill this void in my life."

I was really reaching out to God—searching for more of Him. Blessed by being raised in a Christian home, I grew up knowing that God loved me and took care of me. I played the guitar in church on Sundays during my high school days, and recognized the power and importance of prayer. But here in Quebec City, I sought less confusion and more assurance about His plan for my life. Today, I realize that God has always had me in the palm of His hand, and that I needn't have felt burdened about what was ahead. However, working through these emotions and thoughts made me realize that my relationship with God had been at a standstill. It would, however, take major leaps and bounds over time into a realm of faith and trust in Him.

When I thought of Gary, there was always a special feeling and a question mark within my heart. I had a picture taken of the two of us lifeguarding at Maple Grove Park which sat in a frame atop my dresser in my room at Ste-Foy, Quebec. Once a friend questioned me about the picture. "Who is that nice looking man with you?"

"Just a good friend," I casually replied.

"Only a friend?"

"That's all." I couldn't say more than that because, frankly, I didn't know where I stood with him. His world was one of university, swimming and travel. *Did he have room for me?* I didn't know. Maybe friendship was all he could offer anyone.

The following summer I was to question our relationship even more. We dated frequently, bonding in our appreciation for music and outdoor beauty. We attended outdoor plays at Malkin Bowl in Stanley Park and shared dinners, picnics, the theatre and concerts. Being in his company was so enjoyable to me. He was sincere, bubbly, lovable and thoughtful. *The man has a heart of gold,* I thought. *But, has he truly captured my heart?* Although I admittedly craved being committed to one person, I was not at all sure that this would be possible with Gary. I did feel safe in accepting him as a true, committed friend. Once, after Gary had hurt my feelings, I returned home after work to find a dozen red roses welcoming me at my doorstep. There was a note:

> Christine, sometimes when I try so hard, I fail. This time I failed. I want to explain, but don't know if I can. Thank you for giving me the most wonderful summer of my life. I do love you in a very special way—wish I could tell you. Love G.

I felt so deeply for Gary but I wasn't really his girlfriend. *Perhaps,* I thought, *I was trying too hard to make the relationship work.* This just brought me pain. *That's it,* I told myself, *I will try to put in my mind that we are friends, and I will expect nothing more.*

At last it was graduation day! Gary and I graduated on separate days in May of 1985. He with a Bachelor of Education Degree and myself with a Bachelor of Arts, majoring in French. I gave him a picture of me clad in cap and gown and grin, knowing that I was going to spend several months traveling in Western Europe. He seemed appreciative and I found out later that my grad picture adorned his fridge while I was away.

Gary and I went out the night before I left Vancouver. "You're excited about this trip, aren't you?"

"Yes, I am. I'm sure you understand, seeing how you are the seasoned traveler."

"I hope you have a wonderful time. Be sure and keep a

journal."

Was it my imagination or did he seem to be uneasy about my leaving?

"Oh, Christine," he teased. "You're going to fall in love and come back married to someone from Europe."

"Not likely Gary. I'm not on that kind of search. I'm not traveling to create ties." *Not, new ties,* I thought.

When we parted, there was no heart-wrenching emotional struggle. Just a temporary good-bye between two close friends. I would be back in December and, in the meantime, we both promised to write.

Write? Well, Gary not only wrote letters, but novel-like descriptions of the latest happenings at Maple Grove Park. He filled me in on who was new on staff, how the kids had grown, his upcoming competitions and travel, and how he missed me being there. "Working at Maple Grove Park is not the same without you," he wrote. My heart danced but then I remembered my promise not to be hurt again. *Just friends, Christine. Just friends.* Admittedly, though, I looked forward to his letters arriving at my grandmother's house near Chartres. Two or three times Gary even telephoned. Elated, I thought, *I must be very dear to his heart.*

Once he called me from Germany with a request: "I'm in Frankfurt. Can you please come to Fulda? It's really close to Frankfurt. I'll be there for a whole week."

I felt torn. "It's really tempting, but I can't."

"Oh, come on."

"Gary, I would love to see you but I have a job lined up that very same week in Reims."

"What kind of a job?"

"I'll be picking grapes in the heart of the champagne region."

He was disappointed, but the timing really was too short. It could not have worked. Weeks later another phone call reached my grandmother's home—this time from Vancouver.

She came running out to find me.

The tone of his voice told me that something was wrong. This was puzzling since he was home from Germany and had a teaching job lined up in Los Angeles. This had been firmed up in the summer.

"I had my car jam-packed, after putting all other belongings in storage," he explained. "Your bike rack was attached to my Volkswagen and I was ready to leave, then I decided to check my mail one final time."

"And? Gary, tell me what's wrong!"

"There was a letter from the Los Angeles school district informing me that my contract had been cancelled."

"Oh Gary, I'm so sorry. I don't know what to say."

"Christine, how could this happen? Where do I turn now? What should I do? My plans are shattered."

Comforting him as best I could, I offered, "I'm sure that another door will open. Don't panic. It will all work out. I wish I could give you a hug."

Later, I learned that he had hung up the telephone and, in anger, with frustration and tears, took a long walk along the beach, deciding to put his faith elsewhere. Buying a newspaper, he searched the ads and applied with the Campbell River School District for a job in high school special education. Although his training dealt primarily with art and art therapy, he did have a few courses in special education, as well as a tremendous amount of practical experience. He decided it was worth a try. A district representative immediately responded to his inquiry with a telephone call. "Can you come for an interview?" he asked eagerly.

Gary was greeted at the ferry terminal and had the interview in the front seat of a station wagon. An offer was made and the contract signed on a handshake. Then, going back to his basement suite, he repacked a few things and attempted a second move—this time to Vancouver Island. This move was to last the year.

When I received a letter from him, his words made me cry with joy. "Christine," he wrote, "I never was a strong believer in God although I knew there was something; but you know, and now I know, that He exists. Everything was planned beautifully, even though I could not see the light . . . everything turned out perfectly."

Thus began Gary's route to knowing God in a personal way.

When I returned home from Europe just before Christmas, I began to knit a sweater for Gary. *Did I want to be hurt? No! Did I like him? Yes! Did I love him? I couldn't or wouldn't allow myself to answer this question.* Anyway, I hoped he would appreciate this homemade gift and, since timing was rather crucial, I sent him a ball of wool with a note that read, "present to follow." I sent him the finished product sometime in March and he loved it. Probably because he, too, always took the time to make gifts, wrapping them in unique ways and stuffing them with love. My gift showed him that I cared.

I decided to continue my education the following September in a French Immersion Training Program at the University of British Columbia. In the meantime, I was employed at the France Pavilion for the duration of Expo 86, as well as as the BC Automobile Association in the Membership Services Department, and at the Red Cross as a telephonist. Needless to say, I was busy. Gary, during this time, was still teaching in Campbell River, venturing over to Vancouver occasionally for swim meets.

When he was in town one weekend, he called to make arrangements to meet on Friday night, however, he never called back to confirm. On Saturday he called again, this time to say, "The team is getting together again somewhere this evening. I'll call to confirm the time and place."

"Sounds great. I'd love to see you."

He never did call. I began to lose faith in this man that I

cared so much about.

Is he for real? I asked myself. *Is this how you treat a best friend? Why was he leading me on in such a cruel way?*

Instead of bottling up my hurt, I wrote to Gary, and said I wanted to know where his priorities stood. "Are they with swimming or with me?" I asked. "If I don't have a place, I understand, but I don't appreciate being led on." After mailing the letter, I didn't hear from him for a long time. Later, he explained that my letter made him believe that I didn't really care for him. How confusing!

Working at Expo 86 was a great experience and a place where I made lifelong friends. Although I saw Gary once or twice on the site, there was no communication during that period. Once again I was trying to forget about my attachment to him. The more I tried to be involved, the more I got hurt. No way did I need this heartbreak!

With God's help I juggled my academic year, working two jobs. Hindsight is always revealing and I now realize that had Gary been in my life at that time, something would have suffered: jobs, relationship, or education. Instead, while my concentration was on studies, I continued to keep tabs on Gary—in both his swim travels as well as his teaching career.

Gary moved back to the Lower Mainland where he taught in Abbotsford—again with special needs students in the high-school setting. He loved his job and built up a superb program. One of the teaching assistants who worked with him was extremely supportive, dynamic and a real witness to Gary's increasing faith in God. When he arrived at school, bubbling with questions about Christian values, biblical stories and God, his friend guided him through some of the answers.

As a student in the teaching profession, I thought it would be interesting to go out and observe Gary and his class.

In all honesty, it was a good excuse to visit with a dear friend.

There I met his classroom assistant whom I had heard so much about. She and I chatted while he conducted an integrated physical education class. Looking back, I realize that Gary had obviously talked with her about the two of us. She drilled me with questions about our relationship and my future goals.

Slowly, the wheels of love began to turn again. Perhaps they had never really stopped. Since the moment I had first met him, this man had always been on my mind. It made me extremely happy that he continued in his search for a deeper understanding of God.

May your roots go down deep into the soil of God's marvelous love; and may you be able to feel and understand . . . And so at last you will be filled with God Himself.

Ephesians 5:14-19

"I have loved you with an everlasting love. I have drawn you with a loving-kindness."

Jeremiah 31:3

Chapter Seven

Our Quest for God

Expressing my thoughts in a journal has always been important to me. Some of the entries made after September 1986, when Gary came back into my life, show how confused I felt about him and our "on and off" relationship. I wrote, "It is no longer worth the effort; I would be better off trying to put him out of my mind, to forget . . . "

Never knowing where I fit in, and not wanting to be hurt, even unknowingly, I tried to be indifferent. *Christine,* I told myself, *don't put your emotions at risk!* Friendship? Love? Whatever my fascination with him could be called, I was tired of trying to understand the "why" of it. Because this question dwelled too much in my spirit, my heart was heavy. And so my feelings for Gary were kept in check by closing the door to my inner, deepest emotions. Although, I cared deeply for Gary, I wasn't sure if such feelings could be described as love.

Besides, even the dearest of friendships, needed to be honestly defined to be understood and enjoyed. And so, whenever I saw Gary, a part of me remained detached. Later, I was to understand that these were not easy times for him. As he grew spiritually, he was also addressing confusing issues in regard to his identity and life-style.

In February of 1987, Gary finally began disclosing matters close to his heart. We were having dinner at a quaint restaurant to celebrate my birthday. "Christine, I know that we haven't seen much of each other over the past year. I also realize that, in the past, I hurt you by what appeared to be indifference, but," he said, stopping to drink a sip of water, "I want you to know I have been walking closer with God."

"That's wonderful," I replied, wondering where he was going with the conversation.

"All of my life I've had this empty feeling inside, but God has filled the emptiness. He's given me a true identity— a new strength."

"He is the only one who can fill our needs," I added. "I, too, did a lot of searching before I realized this."

As we sat there discussing who God is and how He changes our lives, I felt joy for this new assurance that Gary had found. He spoke of regrets for past behavior but rejoiced in the knowledge that he was forgiven.

I smiled. "We have all been down the road of regrets, but a new road has been paved."

Then we talked about our relationship. "You've always been very dear to me, Christine. My feelings for you go way beyond friendship."

I tried to be honest. "I've always had deep feelings for you, too." *Careful, Christine,* I told myself. *Don't open the door too wide, too fast.*

Through tears, he shared some more. "I never dreamed that the feelings I had for you would be reciprocated. I do love you."

46

But, I thought, *is the love strong enough to give me a place in your life? Do you love me as a close friend or as a woman with whom you want to share a commitment?* I was afraid to grow too attached to him, not wanting to be vulnerable to the same kind of heart-wrenching pain I had experienced before.

For the next several days, I did a lot of thinking. I re-read the correspondence that Gary had sent to me over the years. There was the "novel" he wrote to me when I was in France—and the long distance phone calls from Vancouver, Germany. Even with such displays of affection, I didn't know if we had anything more than a friendship. I had invested much energy and emotion in this relationship. *Was it paying off? Dare I open my heart to further risk? We both needed time to grow in our walk with God while we dated, laughed, and cried together.*

A year later I was a first-year teacher, honestly wondering why I was working so much, being at school at 7:00 a.m., leaving after 5:00 p.m., only to cart boxes of books and papers home to mark, lessons to plan, report cards to prepare. As the months trudged by, things got a bit easier for me, and there was light at the end of the tunnel. Though the job was exhausting, I was happy with the school year and looked forward to my next class. God would see me through anything.

Being relatively new to the Christian faith, Gary would ask questions and stir up conversation that would get me thinking and questioning my own beliefs and values. Being brought up in a Catholic family didn't automatically put me on the exact path God wanted me to follow. I, too, needed to seek His will for my life. Unsure about my future or what I wanted in life, I turned it over to God. He would be my guide.

When Gary came to take me out, he would have a smile on his face and flowers in hand, much to the delight of my three roommates—and me. *But, was he to be a part of my life? Could I ever again fully open that door to my heart?*

With God, anything is possible, I told myself. *But be cautious.*

Gary often loaned me tapes of Christian music which we sometimes listened to as we traveled in the car. Also, we talked about the Bible and shared more and more about God. Our faith became part of us and we began to build upon this foundation. One day Gary told me about a great little church he had stumbled upon. "Will you join me one Sunday, Christine? I think you'll like it. The singing is uplifting and inspiring."

Without hesitation, I agreed. "I'd like very much to go."

As church became a part of our week's activities, sometimes I would go my own way, and he, his way. Frequently, we would connect.

One Sunday morning in March of 1988, Gary openly conveyed that God was in His life by being baptized with his family and mine present. That same day, he gave this testimony:

> As I stand here today, I can't help but think of the thousands of events that took place during my pilgrimage. I often compare my pilgrimage to the life of a 2-year-old boy who has just learned to run—usually in the opposite direction of his parents.
>
> For most of my life, I, too, was that small boy running in opposite directions, finding dead end roads and paths that lead to nowhere. The Lord was constantly tugging on my ear, pulling me back, trying to open my eyes to the Spirit, but . . . I just didn't listen and I just couldn't see.
>
> There were many events in the past 2 years that opened my eyes, but one particularly that I would like to share.
>
> I was conducting a physical education class at the high-school I worked at—we were playing basketball. My attention was continually being focused on a young lady who seemed to possess a gift for basketball. She could set up and dunk a basket with amazing agility. It

wasn't only her physical talent that caught my attention, but the whole spirit in which she moved.

She seemed so light and so full of joy, every play was with such supernatural talent. I knew she was a Christian; and I knew that what I had witnessed was not just an extremely talented basketball player, but what I saw was a person who was filled with the Holy Spirit.

I suppose it wouldn't even matter if she could play basketball at all, she walked in the spirit and the spirit walked in her.

My eyes seemed to open and I began to understand what a powerful, wonderful and joyous life it could be if you let the Holy Spirit in.

I drove home that day, crying most of the way, asking the Lord to continue His work with me and that some day, I, too, would be filled with the Holy Spirit.

I've come a long way since then, this only illustrates one of the many events that helped me during my pilgrimage.

My ears seem to hurt less these days, and my eyes see a lot clearer. Again I see myself as that two-year-old boy filled with energy and ready to run . . . but this time, I've got a wonderful Light to guide me.

This marked the beginning of something greater. Gary and I began to go to church together, varying the location from time to time. Just as Gary was delighting in the realization of God's presence, I, too, felt a surge of renewed assurance and optimism about the future. God was very much a part of our lives. My "if only he believed in God" of yesterday had became the reality of today.

Although I continued to ask questions and wondered if I would ever be ready for a lifetime commitment to this man, I trusted that God would give me answers in His time. With Him as our common ground and our Rock, our love was becoming deeper and more focused.

God was leading Gary to Him and, ultimately, to me. The quest for God in our lives as a couple crescendoed.

*Dear friends, let us love one another, for love comes from God . . .
since God so loved us, we also ought to love one another.*

1 John 4:7, 11

"No one has ever seen God; but if we love one another, God lives in us and his love is made complete in us."

1 John 4:12

Chapter Eight

Interlude on a Starlit Night

Scrawled out in the center of a huge piece of pink poster paper taped haphazardly to a wall for a party my roommates and I had, were these words: "Christine, when you see a falling star, then it will start to happen. G."

It was our graffiti wall and, amidst notes and comments from all sorts of people, this one shone. Over morning coffee the day after the party, I could not help but smile when I saw the note.

What, I wondered, *will start to happen? What did I want to happen?* When cleaning the room, I carefully ripped out that section, safely tucking it away in my journal.

Dinner at an exquisite West Vancouver restaurant on a starlit night provided an elegant prelude to strolling along the pier, looking for the few constellations we were capable of identifying in the speckled sky. Gary broached the topic of falling stars, determined to see one that night.

"Maybe we'll see one . . ." he mumbled.

In reply, I asked, "Isn't it when you are looking for something in particular that it hides? Come on, it's May. The chances of spotting a falling star are pretty slim. The meteorites are most prevalent in August when the earth is nearest the meteorite shower."

He looked at me somewhat puzzled. "You sound like an expert."

"I am—sort of. My brothers, sister and I used to camp out in our back yard the nights of August tenth or eleventh. We stayed up as late as we wanted, just to see the shooting stars. Can you imagine five kids all shouting at once? 'I saw one! I saw another one! Did you see that one?' " I chuckled at the fond memories.

Although Gary smiled and appeared happy, he was also quiet and rather pensive. How was I to know that he had other things on his mind!

There is something very wonderful about receiving personal mail or notes on a special occasion. Gary often left notes on my car on his way to swim practice, well before I was ever acquainted with the day. Sometimes there were flowers for my desk at school. The last week of June 1988, I received a hand painted dinner invitation in the mail. Gary always made his own cards—a craft I adopted, too, later on. The card was decorated with a charming, romantic table setting for two, a dinner date reserved for the first of July, which was the first day of summer holidays. It read, "You are invited to a very special celebration in your honor."

Wondering what I had done to deserve all of this, I graciously accepted.

Gary arrived right on time, laden, as always, with flowers in hand. At Sprinkler's Restaurant in Vandusen Gardens, the summer night eavesdropped on us as we chatted about our friendship, our separations, our reunion, and our God.

We believed that God had continuously put us together and that He had a plan. Admittedly, I liked the way things were going, and something inside me began to respond. This wasn't the past. We were both traveling a new road.

When the restaurant was almost deserted, Gary reconfirmed his love for me over and over again and expressed how grateful he was to God for our relationship. "I think it appropriate," he shared excitedly, "that I give you a little present. Here Christine, something for you to celebrate."

"Shall I guess?" I asked, expecting one of his inspiring paintings or a unique drawing.

"Sure, go ahead, but it's different from anything I have ever given to anyone before."

The way it was wrapped I was sure it was a drawing; however, instead of guessing, I opened it, carefully and slowly.

Gary had written and illustrated a poem for me. *Come Again* was composed from the depths of his heart; and, as I read it, I knew that I no longer needed to hold back for fear of being hurt. I loved Gary and was ready to make a commitment. Six months prior I would not have been ready to do so. To this day, I treasure the poem:

Come Again

Come Again
Her open hands stretched out to me even as I rebelled
And filled my soul with pride
Those rebellious days turned into years and my
Heart slowly drifted into darkness

Come again
let me feel the light of your heart upon my face
let us dance with the heavens to the beat of the stars
Come Again

In my darkness, her light never dimmed
As the comfort of her hands stretched even further

Finally, my pride crumbled and I fell to the
Ground only to be caressed by the rays
Of her love . . .

Come again
let me feel the light of your heart upon my face
let us dance with the heavens to the beat of the stars
Come again

As my broken body lifts from the ruins of pride,
She waits,
Patiently, and lovingly
Enduring my cross and soothing my wounds
With her open hands

Come again
let me feel the light of your heart upon my face
let us dance with the heavens to the beat of the stars
Come again,
Come again.

For Christine
With unconditional love
And God's blessing,
Gary

`,,,,,,,,,,,`

After indulging in dessert and coffee, we left the restaurant, hand in hand, strolling toward the car. It seemed to be misting out; but we soon realized that this mist was a distant sprinkler, adding droplets to a romantic interlude.

Do I still have to wait for a falling star to ask you to marry me?

"No," I whispered, then added, "but when?"

"Well, not tomorrow," he whispered lovingly in between 'I love you,' smiles and hugs. I knew that I was going to marry my best friend. Other sprinklers near us, with their fine spray, reminded us of the play *Singing in the Rain* that we had seen at Malkin Bowl years previously in Stanley Park. Upon leaving, we had gotten soaked. It seemed as though history had just repeated itself.

The next few weeks our conversations revolved around where we would marry, when, and whom we would invite. It was thrilling to have Gary introduce me as his fiancée—a long-awaited dream. We kept the engagement quiet for a month, since we wanted to look for a ring together and then surprise everyone. It wasn't easy to contain the smiles, the joy and the happiness I was experiencing. We vowed our path would be the one alongside God, for we would need Him to grow in faith and in His love. We had come a long way as a pair. How I thanked the Lord then, and continue to do so today. Because we wanted a summer wedding, we set the tentative date as July 8, 1989, a year away. Gary still had swimming competitions left, including the Paralympics in Seoul, Korea; therefore, it would simply be too rushed and stressful to try and plan it any sooner.

When summer drew to a close, Gary was getting ready to go to Holland for his final training camp before going to Seoul. It had been a wonderful summer spent together with friends. Now it was time to prepare for our respective classes in the fall.

A friend loves at all times . . .

Proverbs 17:17a

"Your love has given me great joy and encouragement . . ."

Philemon 7

Chapter Nine

Planning a Wedding

The months following our engagement, after the diagnosis, were colored with pain, sadness, joy and encouragement wherever we went. Through prayer, faith in each other, and the support of others, we were able to bridge the uncertainties of AIDS and enter into the certainty of God and His faithfulness. Yes, AIDS was a reality but so was God.

Knowing that we now had the support of both of our families, we began planning our very special day—the one that was to mark a lifetime of commitment, trials, tribulations, and love. To this very day I feel blessed and would make the same decision over again—that of marrying my best friend regardless of the fact that he had AIDS.

Perhaps one might think that life would have been easier had this not been our choice. This is not true! Had we given up our dream, what would have happened to the hope and zeal we had for life? We would have missed the joy and jubilation of sharing our lives together in a union that allowed our love to become deeper and richer. By sharing the good and the bad, we experienced God's grace, His love, and His compassion in a supernatural way.

Gary and I were teammates in planning the wedding, sharing ideas and then putting them into action. Although it was time-consuming, we found much pleasure in making our wedding invitations. We had tentatively booked a hall months previously, but when we got a call saying that someone else wanted the location for the same day, we let them have it. That was the deciding factor that our wedding reception would take place in my parents' backyard—west coast weather permitting. An outdoor reception among flower beds and trees would be a living reminder of the Creator and His workmanship.

Like most brides-to-be, I was bombarded with questions about the wedding. "What is your dress going to be like? When are you going to get it? Who will you have in your wedding party? What colors will the wedding party wear? What about a bridal registry?" This was all exciting but I couldn't help but think how trivial it was compared to the emotional challenges we had already faced and those that still lay ahead of us. What really mattered to us was that we would finally be united in God's name.

Gary and I had been to eleven weddings in 1988 and we joked about taking notes at all of them. Then I was off to Juarez, Mexico to see one of my brothers marry his Mexican fiancée. Ripping hand-made little hearts and squares out of paper for our wedding invitations made the flight seem short. Of course, it would have seemed even shorter had Gary been at my side; however, he was not able to attend.

It was important to me to write a few letters of reassurance to relatives explaining our situation. I hoped and prayed that they would understand and accept us for our decision, not feeling that I had been "trapped" into marriage. Ultimately, because there is so much fear and misunderstanding of what AIDS is about, many out-of-town relatives chose not to attend the wedding. There were many bumps in the road we had chosen, primarily concerning people from whom we could not feel true support. However, Gary and I prayed together that God would teach us how to respond to these people and situations in exactly the right way—His way.

Realizing that marriage preparation involved not just the wedding day, but the planning of a life together, Gary and I became involved in a weekend retreat called "Engaged Encounter." This was a program initiated by the Catholic Church for couples planning to marry.

Rather leery and hesitant at first about being "preached at," it was Gary who was the most laudatory about the program. Invited guests would talk about various issues, then the engaged couples went off to write letters to each other. Through this exercise, we realized that we were truly "in sync." We grew closer as one in the Lord and prayed that this would continue along the road ahead of us—a road we knew that would have potholes, turns, and dead ends. This "Engaged Encounter" program freed us from a tunnel of tumultuous events so that the true wedding plans could begin. All heart, all soul!

In talking with friends about wedding preparations, I learned that stress often caused a breakdown in communications and also caused hurt feelings. Gary and I were determined that this was not going to happen with us. Although it frustrated me when complaints about doing the programs emerged (it was a tedious task, performed on a hot day, with a not-so-efficient photocopy machine), we succeeded and all cards turned out well. We even managed to make a scroll, printed with our vows, to be given out with the cake.

Having vowed to live a stress-free month of June, I tried to sound enthusiastic when my mother suggested we go "look" at bridal gowns. It was difficult for me to visualize myself in fancy lace, beads, and flowing fabric which, unfortunately, was usually polyester.

"You know," I said thoughtfully, hoping for a positive response, "I'd really like to find a pattern and make my own dress."

My mother was insistent. "At least try on some styles."

So off we went, trying to find some simple gowns for me to try on. There just weren't any that I liked. Finally, after a full day of searching, we did find a simple elegant white dress at a shop downtown, but it wasn't the right length. There I was in the change room of this small boutique, pencil and paper in hand, trying to sketch this dress. I really liked the style, and it was made of cotton. I knew I could make it.

"How about going to the fabric store down the street?"

Mother succumbed to my wishes, not knowing what she was getting into when she found the gorgeous swiss cotton tucked away. But, I think she realized that when buying a wedding dress, it takes months to order it and only then did fitting adjustments take place. I had about six weeks.

The saleslady was most helpful with suggesting how much fabric I would need after examining my tiny scrawled out sketch. With the sale made, we were off and I was happy. *Won't Gary be surprised,* I mused.

Later, Gary asked curiously, "Did you find a dress?"

"Yes, and I think you'll like it." I knew he would like the material because he had been with me in the same store months earlier when I was looking at fabrics.

He had picked out a beautiful blue-green design and had encouraged me to purchase it. "Great for a sundress, Christine!"

Declining, I had said, "It's too expensive." That same fabric, minus the colored motif, was the one my mother and I discovered that day.

Moving in with my parents for the month had seemed practical since my roommates had all found new places to live and Gary and I wouldn't be in Vancouver for the summer. It was a perfect situation, giving me a place of storage for my belongings and easy access to a sewing machine at any time of the day or night! We had to pack for our trip to France prior to the wedding as we were scheduled to leave two days after the ceremony.

Apparently Gary didn't have one suspicion about me making my wedding dress. When he asked for details about it, my responses were vague—after all, the dress wasn't made yet.

Once, when we were at my friend's family cabin in Sechelt, her mother almost gave the secret away. "How's the hem coming along on your dress, Christine?"

Wide-eyed, I looked at Gary, who seemed absorbed in his own thoughts. Quickly I changed the subject and the question was forgotten.

The day before the wedding, I fastened the bow to my dress. It was ready. The time for our dream to become a reality had come.

Love . . . always protects, always trusts, always hopes,
always perseveres. Love never fails.

1 Corinthians 13:7-8a

*"Marriage is not measured in moments of time,
but in timeless moments."*

Christine and Gary
July 8, 1989

(cross-stitched by one of Gary's students)

Chapter Ten

Best Friends—God Unites Us

Although I don't have a photographic memory, I will never forget the beautiful expression on Gary's face when I was joyfully walking down the church aisle. This moment in time is forever etched in my memory. Recognizing the familiar fabric, he leaned over to say, "You *made* your dress! *When* did you have the time?"

I smiled. "No problem." Inwardly, I thought, *God provided the time. It had all worked out perfectly with no stress. And Gary loved the dress as I had known he would.*

Our wedding day was truly blessed. I awoke early to cloudy skies, but with so much sunshine in my spirit, I couldn't be upset about anything. Later in the day, God's sunshine would pour down upon us; and, in the meantime, nothing could dampen my spirits.

People commented on how calm we were. Our attitude of "why be stressed when it is so exciting and such a happy time" seemed to satisfy most people's curiosity. Having been through months of draining and tense times, this was to be the most joyful of celebrations. Gary and I were overjoyed to have made it to this day. Despite minor problems like forgetting bouquets for flower girls, the ceremony truly celebrated God in our lives. We had put so much forethought into all the planning of our wedding.

Gary walked up the aisle first with his mother and father beside him; I followed suit with my parents beside me. It was difficult to believe that the two of us were finally getting married. Gary looked magnificent and his eyes conveyed tenderness. I was home.

Prior to our wedding, Gary and I had discussed music and I was getting caught up in what songs I wanted played. We could not come to a decision and this really bothered me. Finally, Gary reassured me, "Christine, just leave the music to me; trust me."

And so I did, knowing that we had similar tastes; it was a relief just to turn it over to him. Gary did not disappoint me; the music was wonderful. There were medleys of all the songs we loved and talked about as well as a very special surprise for this celebration. Gary wrote the lyrics and a friend composed the music to the following song:

My Friend

Christine my friend, your love has filled my heart
Christine my friend, you were meant to be a part of my life
and my days,
Even when I walked away
You were right there for me,
Now I am here for you today.

You came again and let me feel
The light of your heart upon my face

Christine my friend, my lover, you and me
Christine my friend, God has chosen you to be
The one to share my joy, the one to share my pain
Sometimes it may be hard, but He is with us all the way.

You came again and let me feel
the light of your heart upon my face
O let us dance with the heavens to the beat of the stars;
Then together we will always be
Forever in eternity
Praising Him who is worthy
The Father of our souls.

Christine
I'll always love you
Be by your side
My best friend
My bride.

The words that Gary had created spoke deeply to the heart. When we were discussing this later, Gary admitted, "I didn't always know how to show my love to you. I wanted this song to make you understand how I feel."

"You've always been original and creative," I replied, but this song has outdone everything."

After exchanging vows, the priest sent us off with the affirmation to go have fun, always be friends, and to continue to open our home and hearts to hospitality. We made our way to my parents' backyard beauty where we celebrated with family and friends.

The tables Gary and I had rolled out onto the lawn the day before were now dressed with linens; and friends welcomed us to a gorgeous backyard reception. Having most of one's family and friends in one place at one time is an incredible feeling. We were the common link to all of these people. We were spellbound with their presence, sharing our day. The wedding vows we had photocopied and rolled into small scrolls were given to each guest with a piece of cake. The words are forever inscribed in my heart:

> With my heart, I will honor God above all
> As I know God will honor me in the joining of our lives.
> As we grow together, sharing in all that our God gives us,
> I look forward to the challenges, the joys and the love
> that He has promised
> In both times of happiness and times of sadness.
> My commitment to you is that of unconditional love from
> this moment forth.
> My faith is in God's hands, and my hope in our future.

Friends roasted us, we laughed hard, a fire was lit in the barbecue pit where night lovers danced and sang . . . we did the garter thing, chatted more, and were finally accompanied by the dozen night owls to our car. We hadn't bothered with going-away outfits. We were clad in our black and white . . .

We drove off in our car, done up with everything imaginable from pie plates, balloons, and shaving cream; confetti flying out of the vents. Stray confetti makes its way out of the vents to this very day. I smile. A happy reminder. What a wonderful world.

What a Wonderful World

I see trees of green, red roses, too
I see them bloom for me and you
And I think to myself
What a wonderful world.

I see skies of blue and clouds of white
The bright blessed days
The colors of the rainbow
So pretty in the sky
Are also on the faces of people going by
I see friends shaking hands
Saying "How do you do?"
They're really saying "I love you."

I hear babies crying
I watch them grow
They'll learn much more than I'll ever know
And I think to myself
What a wonderful world.
Yes, I think to myself
What a wonderful world.

Louis Armstrong

*The Lord is righteous in all his ways and loving
toward all he has made.
The Lord is near to all who call on him, to all who
call on him in truth.
He fulfills the desires of those who fear him; he hears
their cry and saves them.
The Lord watches over all who love him.*

Psalm 145:17-20

"Do not be anxious about anything, but in everything, by prayer and petition, with thanksgiving, present your requests to God. And the peace of God, which transcends all understanding, will guard your hearts and your minds in Christ Jesus."

Philippians 4:6-7

Chapter Eleven

Picture-Perfect Days?

W *ho said dreams never come true?* Our dream of being married was realized. If someone had turned the clocks back to 1982, I would never have imagined such joy and happiness or a love with so much devotion. The happiest day of my life blossomed into a summer of travel with my best friend, complete with camping, morning rituals of café au lait and croissants, winding roads in the French countryside and totalling over 4000 km; the only "pépin" was one flat tire.

We traveled the dream trip of France's country roads together in a new car that Gary creatively described as a glorified lawn mower, packed with camping gear and, of course, swim suits. Our rented, glorified lawn mower had no timetable, no agenda, no itinerary. The only commitment we had was to meet a Swedish friend in Portugal's Algarve at the beginning of August. She had booked her holidays so that we could see her and, as a threesome, we spent a week venturing to some of Portugal's more remote beaches, our trustworthy vehicle leading the way.

My journal entries stopped shortly after our wedding and didn't begin again until the end of February, 1991. My personal entries were inscribed in my heart, in our conversations and in the countless notes and cards we would send to each other via car, mail, or hand delivery.

Gary, however, would occasionally record our adventures and impressions on some of the various trips we made together. Most quoted Scripture in this book is taken from cards we wrote and sent to each other over the years.

Staying healthy for the duration of the trip was what one would have called a mini goal; however, for us it was a major hope. It was one of our greatest prayers. We had the names of doctors in both Paris and in Arles for routine bloodwork; we also had a listing of reputable doctors in the event of a true emergency. The doctors who arranged for the bloodwork were very kind, but the tests often took longer than anticipated. Because we were so used to the efficiency of our health care system at home, this was a source of some stress.

At times my thoughts became the enemy. *What if Gary got really sick? What would I do?* Knowing where the nearest hospital was situated was a part of my hidden agenda. "Lord," I would pray, "please protect us." Instantly, I would feel comforted.

These months were our first time to be constantly together. As any traveler knows, spending twenty-four hours together can sometimes be trying. I was being acclimatized, not only to our rainless summer, but also to Gary's mood swings. At times it seemed as though our common desire to know one another through and through caused us to stumble. This, in turn, only drew us nearer to our Rock.

"We didn't leave all our problems back in British Columbia," Gary commented.

I agreed. "That's true. We are both dealing with intense emotions."

"How could anyone love me?" he asked. "I've made such mistakes—now you are suffering because of them."

"How could anyone not love you? I committed to this marriage because you are the man I deeply love."

"There's . . . there's so much I regret. I keep remembering—"

"God doesn't remember. He says our sins are buried at the bottom of the sea."

Sometimes when Gary was feeling very low, I knew he needed space. Respecting this desire was not always easy because I wanted to be there for him. "Please, tell me what you are feeling, Gary."

"I can't, Christine. Not now!"

"But you taught me to express myself, to tell you how I feel. When I don't, you get frustrated with me. Can't you understand that I feel the same way?"

"Yes, but I'm the one who has . . . has . . . " Not finishing the sentence, he simply mumbled, "I need to be alone for awhile."

And so I would give him his quiet time.

Yes, we had our quarrels, but they were never quarrels of hate or anger; they stemmed from frustration arising from the lack of communicating.

Although most of my relatives live in France, we decided that we would not visit any of them. An authentic visit with my family would mean spending at least half of our eight-week holiday immersed in family formalities and gatherings. And to be truthful, we had experienced some hesitancy and reluctance within the family to see us. *It wouldn't be fair to put Gary through that,* I told myself. It seemed that in France I was very emotional about "us."

Every so often, Gary would ask, "What about the future, Christine? Yours? Mine?"

Although I tried to be encouraging, my mind, too, silently echoed these thoughts. *Would we ever celebrate a wedding anniversary?* As each married relationship is unique, our union was like none other.

There were other questions asked that replayed in our own minds. *How can you bear to be so much in love, and yet not be able to have children? Isn't it impossible for you to express your love fully and freely in intimacy? Christine, aren't you afraid of getting AIDS? Gary, aren't you afraid of giving her AIDS?*

Living in the intimate contacts of marriage, we had to ensure that I would not contract HIV. There are no prophylactics that guarantee 100 percent safety from contracting the virus. Abstinence is the only thing that could give such a guarantee. We had to be careful, responsible, and make sacrifices. Our sexual relationship was not the focus of our love and, therefore, not the central hardship in our married life. There is no denying that it was extremely difficult, very frustrating, and emotionally painful to deal with our sexual limitations; however, our love was so deep, and so committed on a spiritual level that, with God's strength, we were able to cope, and able to experience the other's love both emotionally and physically.

When Gary was diagnosed with AIDS, the news turned our lives around forever. Gary and I knew we would never experience the joy of maternity and paternity together. This, too, stung. I remembered the words that Gary had written to me while I was in France: "I guess we'll be raising our children with the same faith that you've always had, and the new faith that I've accepted." (September 1, 1985)

Chin up Christine, don't lose your hope faith or love—one day we will be free from this . . . for eternity!

Card from Gary—July 10, 1990

"Keep on loving each other as brothers. Do not forget to entertain strangers, for by so doing some people have entertained angels without knowing it."

Hebrews 13:1-2

Chapter Twelve

A Place To Call Home

Soon the trip was over and we were faced with the exciting task of finding a place we would call home. Our home! Having dismissed the thought of purchasing a house, we searched for weeks on end for a small abode on the west side of Vancouver. We had both lived in this neighborhood and loved the character of the homes. The people were friendly and there dwelled a sense of community even within a city. Also, we wanted to remain close to UBC for swimming and potential medical need, should it arise.

People asked why we didn't just buy a house. "Why not move out of the expensive city and put your rent dollars toward a mortgage?" We knew we could not afford the price or the medical cost of time and energy by moving away. Mortgage costs, in our situation, were not our priority at the time.

Only God knew what tomorrow would bring and we did not want to become bankrupt in our spiritual values.

After countless visits to neglected houses with astronomical rent, we had one hope left. Someone had phoned my parents' home over the summer stating that they knew of a family going away for two years. Their house would be available for rent. The only problem was that it would not be available until the end of December. Would we wait?

"Yes! Yes!" we jubilantly answered. It would be worth it since, in all our searching, we had seen nothing to compare with the character, beauty and affordable rent of this house in Dunbar. God had answered our prayers. We would be patient. In the interim, my parents had two boarders, one who was absolutely thrilled to come home to prepared meals, a magnificent garden, and loving in-laws. I, too, was happy, but since I had spent my whole life growing up in these surroundings, it wasn't a novel experience for me. We rented my brothers' old room, were treated like royalty, and Saturday morning breakfasts together were a treat. Gary learned a lot about me through my relating to my family. It was a once-in-a-lifetime opportunity, or challenge, depending on how you looked at it.

Throughout December, we began moving boxes in the basement of the rental house. I would arrive at work with the car loaded to the hilt and, after work, venture off to Collingwood Street. Then it would be home to my parents' house. Just prior to Christmas, we moved into our new rented home. We acquired a sweet, docile dog named Cassie, to whom we became particularly attached, and a cat, Friskie. This was to be our home for the next two years.

With the many changes and adaptations over the first few months in B.C., we were also coping with Gary teaching in a new district and being very unhappy with his job situation. It was not like him to dislike his work. He loved special-needs persons, but was faced with political difficul-

74

ties as well as unclear priorities at the school. His class did not seem to be a priority. With the reallocated budgets, oversized and understaffed classrooms of TMH—trainable mentally handicapped and EMH—educable mentally handicapped—students) waning energy, some weight loss, and the emotional hurdles above and beyond those of this profession; he would come home and break down into tears. Something was clearly not right.

We prayed together for direction from the Lord as to what Gary should do. There was no guarantee of finding another job, unless we were willing to move outside of Vancouver. Medically, this was not feasible. Staying in his present position would only aggravate emotions, alter his positive attitude and, in turn, risk health. We had secured positions in a nearby district in the hopes of eliminating too much commuting. Three years to and from Abbotsford had been enough.

In the beginning of December, Gary and his father were off to Calgary for a four-day visit with his brother. It was a good opportunity for them to spend some time together, as well as a much-needed break for Gary. I was expecting to pick up Gary and his dad at the airport on Monday evening; however, late Sunday night, as I was going downstairs, who did I see walking out of our bedroom, but Gary's father!

My heart sank as I questioned my father-in-law. "What happened?"

"Gary was feeling ill. He got progressively worse so we decided to come home early."

"Where is he?" I asked, my voice quivering.

"In bed."

When I checked on him I didn't like the looks of the situation. "I want to stay home," he insisted. "All I need is some rest." Frightened, I called his doctor, making arrangements for Gary to be admitted to the hospital. I drove him there that night. Later, in his journal, he wrote that, at times, he felt that he just couldn't fight it. He would rather have just gone to sleep forever, but, he wrote, "Christine keeps me alive. She is the reason my heart beats (Well,besides God) . . . I miss her." The doctors eventually diagnosed pneumonia. Fortunately, it was not PCP, but another viral infection that could easily be treated.

Gary was still struggling with what to do about his job. He was definitely not happy with it and felt that the stress at work had contributed greatly to his recent illness. He wanted confirmation from God.

Gary felt that AIDS had taken over his life as indicated by this journal entry. "It controls my eating, sleeping . . . Oh Lord, let You reign, not this disease. It controls Christine, too. Just not fair. Happily they've released me. I can go home today!"

In December Gary finally handed in his job resignation which was accompanied by a report on recommendations for the program's future. He spoke to the administration in the Special Needs Department, and then left on good terms. In January, he began substitute teaching in two districts.

There is something about substitute teaching that makes it very attractive: no report cards, no lengthy staff meetings, no committees, and just short-term planning, if any at all. Gary had such good rapport with children—teenagers in particular. As a teacher on call, he never experienced major disciplinary problems nor the political frustrations of the past.

Because he was happy, I was happy. Not only did this mean he was feeling better, but also that he could substitute in my class while I was away participating in a cultural exchange program. My eight students who were not in the exchange program really enjoyed having their teacher's husband as their substitute.

That same year I was also involved in my school's outdoor education program which meant I ventured off to Vancouver Island with seventy students for five days, minus my husband.

No problem, I thought. *Five days isn't that long.*

I was wrong! The five days seemed like forever and I will never forget my feelings of anticipation when I returned. When the orange school bus dropped me off at a major intersection in Vancouver, I hopped the city transit. Weighed down with my backpack and hiking boots, I felt as though I were traveling the roads of Europe again. With my heart pounding, I hiked the few blocks from the bus stop to our home. Gary was in the kitchen and, when he saw me, the expression of love on his face was so tender. How I had longed for this moment! As we embraced, the surge of heart-felt warmth that welled up was indescribable. There was a renewed bonding of our spirits that gave us an even greater appreciation and understanding of our relationship. Overcome with emotion, we held each other tightly and lovingly, not wanting to ever let go. Never again would we lose sight of the fact that we were each other's priority. This was our precious time together.

As winter blossomed into spring, Gary and I closely observed our garden, noting what came up piercing the earth, and where.

"What do you think, Gary?"

"Looks great, but we need a bit more color. Since you have inherited your father's green thumb, help me decide what to add."

I laughed, "It's only been over the last few years, that this hereditary path finally made its way to me."

"Well, let's see what we can do as a team," he suggested.

And so we planned and planted. One year it was a flower and a vegetable garden, the next year floral beauties prevailed amidst a half dozen tomato plants and one zucchini. Gary regularly cut back the zucchini, fearing it would take up too much flower space.

Color scheming was Gary's forte; he gave me color combinations and, together, we would place the many bedding plants. Because of his weak back, I would do the bending and ultimate planting. We thoroughly enjoyed this team project and revelled in the beauty of its daily outcome. Fresh picked flowers, scented bouquets, and some of nature's truly unique art left our backyard to become beautiful arrangements in the house.

To keep in good physical shape, we continued swimming three times a week with the members of the Masters Swim Club at UBC. Gary swam in lane eight, the fast one, whereas I swam in what some might call the "social" lane. If the conversation at the end of the lap was not compelling enough, swimmers would do tumble turns. When Gary began feeling that he was having a more difficult time keeping warm in the water and ended up in the hot tub sooner than he hoped, we decided to take a break from the swimming, at least for a few months.

Summer melted into fall and with it came a new job for Gary. It was a position in a nearby district which enabled him to work with learning-disabled students. He loved the students and the challenges that he faced in working with them. He cared. Gary, now driven by a job he enjoyed, coped better even with our constant and consistent attention to his health. Of course, there were hurdles and, at times, it felt as though they were strategically placed closer and closer together with barely enough time to get over one, let alone see over it, before there was another.

With every step, however, God was at our side, sometimes guiding us along, sometimes carrying us. The support we experienced from family, friends and our church was immeasurable. Yes, there was still rejection and some situations that proved to be extremely emotional; however, we learned daily how to appreciate what God was giving us. A brand new day! A day together! We would ask ourselves, *What can we do to be more like Him? How can we see Him in the people we meet?* Yes, despite the hurdles, life was wonderful. We were together; we had Him to lean on for strength.

Being with Gary had taught me many things. One of the most obvious lessons was to slow down. As far as walking, I had to "literally" slow down my pace, since Gary was not a power walker. There were times I had to adapt to his new special needs such as the one for more rest. We turned down many invitations to go to dinner or a show, because, if Gary got overtired, the next day would be miserable for him—a write-off. We learned to predict and to accept this. Although I found something beautiful about slowing down, there were times that it weighed heavily upon us. Gary felt so controlled by the disease.

"My illness is hurting both of us," he would say. "It's making us both prisoners!"

"Being with you is what matters," I'd say reassuringly. "I refuse to dwell on anything else. And, besides, most people are aware of our situation."

"And they understand," he'd say thoughtfully. "But what about the ones who don't know the truth? When the time is right, we need to tell them."

"Yes, when we're ready."

A picture-perfect summer day often began with a morning café latté which we would savor in sips, accompanied by a few croissants, on the front steps of our rented house on Collingwood Street. Enjoying the sun's first glow, Cassie, our black lab/terrier would sit near us, ready for any unwanted croissant crumbs and, together, we would greet any neighbors or other persons who passed by. Daily, we watched our flowers grow. Many of our at-home days were spent in our garden—something which surprised my family. They teased me. "Has something happened to our Christine? House plants used to die in her bedroom!"

Not any more, I thought. We plant seeds and then watch them grow into beautiful, creative works of art. Later, I was to learn that we were also planting other seeds that would blossom in the future. They were rich, warm, beautiful memories that no one could ever uproot or take away from me. Happy memories of Gary at the piano, his music, composed in his heart and mind, traveling throughout the house, finding its way outdoors to the back deck where I would be puttering with flower boxes dripping with lobelia and potted geraniums drooping with blossoms. Memories of sound and scent as his music would waft out and mingle with the scent of french lavender. Yes, so many good memories, and more to come.

Now faith is being sure of what we hope for
and certain of what we do not see.

Hebrews 11:1

"But God's truth stands firm. He remains faithful to us and will help us ... and He will always carry out His promises to us."

2 Timothy 2:13

Chapter Thirteen

Depths and Heights

Because of Gary's illness and our desire to fight it together, I gradually became "Nurse Christine." In April of 1990, after a bronchoscopy, Gary was diagnosed with Cytomegalvirus (CMV), a virus that can attack any part of the body. So, when he began having vision problems, he made an appointment with his optometrist. "I'm seeing spots and flashes," he explained. "Something is wrong!"

The doctor made light of his complaints. "Perhaps, you're just getting old?" he said after rushing him through the office visit.

"Getting old," he echoed. "Doctor, I'm only twenty-nine!" Unsatisfied, he searched out a second opinion and was referred to a specialist at St. Paul's Hospital. There the correct diagnosis of CMV was made; but, since the virus had attacked the retina of his right eye, there was little that could be done. We thanked God that he still had his left eye; however, it would have to be monitored very closely.

Treatment for the right eye involved weekly ocular injections of a drug called gancyclovir. Since the eye drops dilated his pupil, blurring his vision for several hours, I drove him downtown. This new treatment became a part of our forever-changing routine. Though I may have felt tired by the strenuous routine, God gave me the strength to handle each new situation calmly and with love. Inwardly, I desired, and was determined to do anything and everything I could to ease the pain, fatigue and frustration that my husband was experiencing. Gary made his final journal entry on October 9, 1990:

> My goal is to keep healthy although sometimes the deterioration of my body consumes my emotions and Christine gets the brunt of it. It is so hard to see my body die—so sad, scary and hurting. The eye injections are going well—I think. There is much to think about; what is God's plan? Lord, we still pray with all our hearts for a cure. Please see us through this trial. Our faith is in you, our love is in you and our hearts cry for your protection.

We walked the hills of life with God, forever trying to catch glimmers of hope. Our minds and hearts were full of questions: *Would the gancyclovir prevent the CMV from affecting Gary's left eye? Was this physical and mental strain of ocular injections worth the results?* A bit of the burden eased when the ocular injections were replaced with intravenous treatment through UBC Hospital's Emergency Ward. As a "regular," Gary always found the staff to be kind and accommodating. He would go for a run of medication before heading off to work, and then again before coming home.

Gary and I, wanting our major commitments elsewhere, fought the idea of being tied down to the hospital. Knowing that he believed his daily treks to the emergency ward were running his life, I tried to be sensitive to his feelings; but it was depressing, and I often felt helpless and frustrated. Yet, in the midst of this depression, I would feel the incredible light of God's presence.

Rejoicing, we thanked God that we were able to free ourselves from the hospital as long as we picked up medication every five days and made sure that Gary's heplock (the needle inserted in the skin on the forearm) was in place and changed on a weekly basis. I had to make special appointments with the nursing staff in order to learn how to administer an intravenous. No longer did we have to stay in the emergency ward to run the medication; instead, I did everything from home. Running the gancyclovir became part of our routine and although it took organization, time, and energy, it was never a bother to me. We would run the intravenous medication twice daily: once before breakfast—prior to me going to work—and again before dinner.

"God," I cried out. "You know how desperately I want everything for my husband. His health. His vision. His carefree spirit." The situations that weighed so heavily on him, also burdened me. *But we were going to make it and we were not going to dwell on the negative. We had to keep our focus on God. His will.*

"But, what is Your will? Give us direction, God." From November 1990 to June of 1991, it became more and more evident that there was something very much the matter with Gary's health. Both of us felt a stronger need to share our story with more people. Gary had a second bronchoscopy in November 1990 which tested negative for PCP. Yet, in January, he began to be increasingly fatigued! In June of 1991, he became blind in his right eye. As indicated by this excerpt from a letter which Gary wrote, our lives continued to be punctuated with hospital stays and new medications:

> My health has been generally good. No major illness except for the loss of my right eye to CMV. I never thought being blind would be so traumatic or emotional, but I accept God's will and if this be His plan, so be it.

To ease the discomfort with the heplock, Gary had a port-a-cath put in over the summer of 1991. I was trained to run the intravenous through this as well. The small device, implanted in the chest, connected a plastic tube with a major vein. The advantage was that the needle, once inserted, could be left in for up to a week, therefore, avoiding too many daily painful attempts at finding the right vein in an arm. Medication was thus pumped from the heart to all parts of the body. We were supposed to run a certain dose over an hour but, admittedly, there were days when we sped it up. Gary tolerated the drug very well; therefore, there was no harm.

Seemingly trivial things were put under a microscope as I learned that small actions could have such a positive or negative impact. Because of Gary's reduced peripheral vision, extra care had to be taken to ensure that the dishwasher and all cupboard doors were closed. Gary would ever so sweetly remind me, in his gentle way. "Christine, you just have to remember to close the cupboards." And I did remember *most* of the time, not wanting a moment of carelessness to be responsible for causing him additional pain.

Despite his visual difficulties, Gary loved to capture the last rays of the sunshine's warmth on the back porch. Moving the potted geraniums to one side, he would lean over the newspaper, trying to read, while enjoying the evening air. This became more painstaking as time went on. On occasion, I read the headlines to him, but soon the newspapers were placed by the fireplace, unread. With shorter days and more medical commitments, there was virtually no time for reading. Trying to focus on the positive, we would enjoy our meals while seated at our outside picnic table as long as the sun's rays would allow. Occasionally we would go out for dinner; however, this, too, became frustrating since restaurant lighting is usually poor. The two of us worked on projects together—homemade presents or an art project on canvas.

Gary gave me advice and suggestions in positioning things in just the right place.

Going away for extended periods of time became virtually impossible. Six days was the maximum we could possibly dream of, and so we were off to the Okanagan Valley to visit some family and friends at Kalamalka Lake. Like a third party, a cooler filled with medication bags, IV tubings, needles, syringes, saline solution, heparin and alcohol swabs accompanied us on our journey.

The myriad of colors shimmering on the sunlit lake seemed to be a reflection of the presence of the glory of God. We stayed with friends whose children constantly brought laughter to the air. They relished Gary's storytelling capabilities, their eager ears and open minds always so ready to capture what the imagination would welcome.

We were able to relax in the summer air; however, it was extremely hot that week, and Gary, who normally enjoyed the heat, found it too hot. He did not venture much past his waist in the lake—almost like Maple Grove Park days—but, instead, rested indoors where it was cooler. He was emotionally and physically drained and his vision was weakening rapidly. When he saw more spots and more flashes, we knew what it meant, and decided to return home earlier than anticipated. We wanted to have things checked out.

The air, already heavy with death-like silence on that ride home, swelled as uncertainties about Gary's vision and future raced through our minds. He was depressed and frustrated at not being able to clearly see the mountains and valleys. Our thoughts and emotions were met with ominous stillness. The depths seemed greater than the heights. For an artist to deal with the loss of vision is like a death sentence in itself. Gary, the painter, always had an eye for beauty whether in nature or in simple things. It seemed so unfair that this was being taken away from him. But, in the midst of this turmoil, there was God, filling our cloudy minds with a reminder that He had a perfect plan for us. We knew that He watched us.

Gary showed me what sight he had by the proximity of the fingers I held in front of his face. It was alarming to see how fast his vision was changing. From morning to night, for two days, there was considerable loss of vision in his left eye. His only good eye was now experiencing a retinal detachment, the tissue having become weakened by the CMV. When it had happened to his right eye, we consoled ourselves, knowing that he still had his left eye. Now, however, our last glimmer of hope was being ripped away. Gary called his opthalmologist on Tuesday morning and saw her at noon, the same day. He was admitted to the hospital for laser surgery on the retina, a peeling, weak tissue that was as rotten as old wallpaper. Eye drops and an eyepatch became part of a more rigid routine in order to prevent infection, to dilate the pupil, and to smooth the healing. This was not accomplished without frustration. I would often close my eyes to try to be where he was, or to squint until all I could distinguish were light and dark, just to get a glimpse of what he was experiencing— a small taste. However, nothing I did could really compare.

"God," I invoked, "I want to help him." But I couldn't take away his pain. All I could do was pray that God's hand would be upon this situation. Waiting for Gary to come out of the operating room, I tried to read the book I had brought with me—also tried to write some letters—all to no avail.

Gary's first words whispered upon recovering from the anaesthetic warmed my heart. "Where am I? Is my wife here?"

Consider it pure joy, my brothers, whenever you face trials of many kinds, because you know that the testing of your faith develops perseverance. Perseverance must finish its work so that you may be mature and complete, not lacking anything.

James 1:2-4

"A cord of three strands is not quickly broken."

Ecclesiastes 4:12b

Chapter Fourteen

Attached by Threads of Love

A nd so another healing process began; it was one that involved God, Gary and me. Perhaps that sounds rather selfish—I don't mean that family and friends didn't count—they did, and I thank God for each and every one of them. They were and are precious, particularly during difficult times. It's just that Gary and I were continually searching for God's will in our lives, for His guidance to find the path He wanted us to take together. We could accept wherever it led, if we were truly in His will.

Here we were dealing with a multitude of uncertainties. *Would his left eye heal? Would he see clearly?* So many unknowns! *Dared we hope that he would ever paint again?* I was afraid of the darkness that was being painted into our lives. Gary was so sick—fighting the loneliness and fear of that darkened world. Though I held and comforted him for better or for worse, prayer was my only weapon to help him fight something that neither of us could fully comprehend.

Would I be able to be strong enough for him? Would I be able to cope with my husband going blind as yet another hurdle being heaped across our path? It seemed impossible. *How will I do it Lord?*

Being physically disabled since childhood, the worst of trials according to Gary would have been blindness. It pained me to think of Gary unable to see, becoming dependent on others, knowing full well that he'd struggled throughout his life to be independent. A handicap he had overcome, but blindness? To have his vision taken away seemed unbearable. *How could God's hand be in this?* We longed to be nearer to God and for Him to be nearer to us. We had to trust. I strongly felt that God, knowing how much Gary would love and appreciate the ability to paint again, would grant him this. We hung on to hope.

"There's a light in our tunnel," Gary proclaimed. "I can see a line, some brightness!"

"How many fingers, Gary? How many do you see?" Nervously, I held my fingers very close.

"Two."

We praised God. At that point, his eye was only partly filled with fluid. The air would diffuse we were told, and the fluid would eventually take its place. Darkness still loomed!

Through my outstretched arms, hugging, tears, and words, I tried to express the love, compassion and empathy I felt for him. With mingling tears and a shaky voice, I reassured my husband. "God is with us, in us, watching us and loving us."

Gary wanted so much to be home with me and, of course, this was also my fervent desire. He was tired and lonely at the hospital. That morning, while alone, he fell against a wall in the bathroom and was hurt. My heart went out to him. How frustrating.

We continued to focus on God's plan, trusting Him and trying to live as though Jesus Christ was our only audience. I wondered, *What are the ramifications of this hurdle?* He knew I never thought of him as a burden, and yet he began asking himself what he would do while I was at work. It had become obvious that he would not be returning to his job.

My sensitive husband had taught me to see beauty in everything that surrounded me, particularly in the symphony of colors alive in our world. Together we learned to appreciate even the most simple things. With Gary being such a visual person, I would momentarily ask how and why God could allow this horrible eye condition to happen. Gary was never one to take his sight for granted. We had once spoken about it.

"Christine, sometimes, I wonder if this is all worth it."

"What do you mean? Don't you think the gancyclovir is working?"

"Look what happened with my right eye. All that I went through and I still lost my vision in just a few months."

I tried to be encouraging. "But Gary, the CMV Retinitis in that eye wasn't detected until it was too late to do much of anything. This is different."

"How?" he asked, his voice very soft. "How is it different? There are still the endless medical appointments of ocular injections and intravenous treatments at home, twice daily. Our lives aren't our own."

"No, they aren't. We belong to God. Hold on Gary, we can make it!"

My words were soon tested. In the fall of 1991, Gary was diagnosed with microbacterium avium infection, a form of tuberculosis. This meant even more medication. Then, not long afterwards, there was the onset of diabetes mellitus. "Most likely, drug-induced," the doctors said. Our morning ritual became more lengthy, adding glucose readings and insulin shots to our regimen. Gary could have administered the insulin himself; however, with his depleting vision, I did it. Anything to make him realize that he was not alone—we were in this battle together.

Toward the end of October, he was diagnosed with aspergillous pneumonia in the lower lobe of the right lung. More medication, including morphine, to ease the pain and discomfort was added to our list. Yes, Nurse Christine was very busy and becoming more knowledgeable about disease and treatment every day.

By September, I noticed that I was not my usual energetic self in the classroom. Although I strived to do my job well and to make myself available to my students whenever they needed me, my heart was at home with my husband. Thoughts of him never left my mind, my soul. I wondered how he was coping and prayed that he would encounter few frustrations. Again, efficient use of breaks and lunch hours enabled me to leave the school as early as possible. Dawdling was no longer in my dictionary and my priorities began to shift yet more. Though I loved my job, I wanted to be at home. We spoke of me taking some time off later in the school year; however, in the meantime, we continued to manage.

That fall Gary and I had a dream that we thought, wondered, and prayed about. It was our prayer and desire that, despite his latest eye problems, he would be able to see well enough to put a paint brush to canvas. Though we knew the probable, bleak outcome in regard to his eyesight, we hung onto our dream and continued to pray. When Gary began to paint on a regular basis, it was truly a labor of love. He painted out of joy though, inwardly, he was in emotional and physical pain. So many paint brushes and canvases were touched by flowers and hearts.

His style had evolved from beautiful abstractions to combinations of color portraying God's beauty around us. Despite the near-blindness, the beauty that he could portray on a canvas was spellbinding. Yes, these were labors of love and patience, filled with thanksgiving to God whose creations we so thoroughly enjoyed and wanted to see captured on canvas.

That fall we lived in our garden and on our deck which was the source of our inspiration. Gary's last series of acrylic paintings were adorned with the vivid black-eyed susans dancing on his canvases. He spent countless hours painting in our basement-studio and, as the weeks wore on, I became his eyes. When he could no longer read the tube to see what color he was using on his canvas, I would step in, comment on how the colors on his canvas blended, and then see him through his finished work. His vision had become so limited that to paint a straight line was extremely difficult, if not impossible. In the end, I signed some of his canvases where he indicated.

When he felt up to it, Gary took the dog for a walk during the day, going around the block, gaining strength and stamina, while desperately trying to use the white cane to his advantage. All other hours of the day, except for my time at school, Gary and I were together with my arm becoming his guide. There were always new challenges which proved extremely frustrating for both of us—watching for cracks in the sidewalk, stopping at curbs, turning a corner, avoiding obstacles, grocery shopping, visiting friends, dinner out. I had become Gary's eyes at all hours. Often, I broke into tears, invisible to Gary, because I had missed an irregularity in the sidewalk, or he had bumped into something, or he simply could not make out what was being served for dinner at a friend's house. It pained him, and me, too. When you feel so much a part of another person, you hurt and grieve for that individual. Feelings of helplessness overwhelmed me.

Prayer had become our strongest link, binding us to one another and to God in a supernatural way. Before bed, holding hands, we would thank God for what He had given us that day. We prayed fervently, with simple words, for His will to be revealed to us clearly, and that He grant us an abundance of strength, courage and wisdom. In the mornings, we had developed the habit of reading from a daily devotional book. As Gary's vision lessened, I would read for both of us. Struggling to overcome the feelings and emotional turmoil while in the valleys of discouragement, we turned to the Lord for help in overcoming the hurdles. With Him and one another, we could do it. Jesus Christ had become the center of our lives, not the background.

In November, we found out that, since our landlords were returning from two years abroad, we would have to leave our quaint rental home. Of course, we'd known that this day would come, but were really hoping that it wouldn't happen until June, after the end of the school year. Once again, we prayed for a home close to the UBC hospital with reasonable rent. But now our requirements were different; we had to keep Gary's depleting vision in mind.

After Christmas, we planned a short holiday to San Diego, looking so forward to some warmth. Gary, particularly, wanted to be in a "bright place." Six days maximum was all we could afford medically. We packed enough medical supplies in a small cooler to take us through one week—we were bound to God, one another, and the supplies in that cooler. Returning just two days before moving day, we were already planning another excursion to Palm Springs for the spring break. It made returning to the classroom easier for me.

Both of us loved the new house we rented. The bathroom that connected to the bedroom was an improvement from the upstairs/downstairs situation on Collingwood. The back deck, too, was a selling rental feature. Already we could visualize the gardening potential which was offered there.

With help from family and friends, we moved all of our belongings the two kilometers from Collingwood Street. It was a difficult time for Gary because he wanted to do much more than he was capable of doing. His vision restricted him.

The settling in process was rather slow and deliberate. It was important to make sure Gary knew where everything was as it was being put away—after all he would be home alone during the day. If Gary was not committed to anything at UBC Hospital, he was at home—facing emptiness and darkness. By himself, he would easily become frustrated and so, after work, I continued to unpack and organize our belongings. My husband, sensitive to the fact that I was also tied to a medical routine of IV's, tried to be considerate of my feelings. He could no longer see well enough to help me with household chores.

After some convincing on his part that I needed a break from some of the home duties, we arranged for a homemaker to come in twice per week. It made a lot of sense to free me from chores so we could spend our precious time together. "Nurse Christine has enough to do," he insisted, firmly but lovingly.

And so, together, we would discuss what needed to be done, and I would prepare a list for the homemaker. With my encouragement, Gary started tape recording his letters to friends, sparing him the frustration associated with trying to write. Every day I would rush home to be with him, treasuring our every moment together. Soon I began wondering if I should even be at work and gently pursued the subject with my husband. "Perhaps you could take a leave of absence the last two months of the school year," he said. "We could do something very special."

We agreed it was something we would definitely think about. "Perhaps we could visit my brother in Mexico," I offered. His smile showed that he liked the idea. It was healing for us to make plans for the future—it gave us something to plan for—to think about.

After being settled in our new home for a couple of weeks, we decided to pay a visit to our former landlords who were staying with friends up the street while the interior of their own house was being repainted. As we headed home after a wonderful visit, Gary made a suggestion: "Let's stop in at the old house and pay Cassie a visit. She's staying there all by herself."

"Great," I said enthusiastically. "We haven't seen her for a couple of weeks."

Creaking open the back gate that rainy night, as though we still lived there, we called out to our dog and, sure enough, Cassie came darting out of the downstairs dog door. She jumped all over us, wagged her tail, and ran circles around the yard.

"She probably wonders where on earth we've been— maybe she's excited about a possible walk!" Longingly, Gary ran his hands over her coat. "Christine, couldn't we take her home, just for one night?"

I hesitated. "Gary, you know our new landlord doesn't allow pets. Tears welled up in Gary's eyes as he struggled with his emotions. Never had we thought a dog could make us feel this way.

At that moment, I felt so very powerless over our situation. Cassie was a pet we both missed, and now that Gary could see so litttle, a companion in the day while I was at work would have been great. As the hinges on the gate creaked behind us, we left, both in tears. Cassie, watching us from the slats of the fence, appeared confused. Her big eyes seemed to say, "They're leaving again. Why are they leaving?" It was the last time Gary saw Cassie.

Gary and I shared so much together—smiles, laughs, despair, happiness, tears and our faith. People even said we looked alike. We also shared our talents with each other, giving the fruit of our labor to one another. Gary gave me treasured moments when he shared art and writing as ways to express his love for me. In return, I made shirts and sweaters for him, finding it fun to try to surprise him with the gifts. Together, both being pianists at heart, we would partake in music and symphonies. Gary often talked about wanting to play the violin in Heaven. Songs and artwork, another bond between us, attached by threads of love, became ever-increasingly more difficult to pull apart.

Because time was precious, we seldom went out without each other. If, at the last minute, Gary felt he could not go somewhere, I would not go either. The few times that I went to functions alone, the circumstances weighed heavily on my mood—whether it was to attend a wedding, a baby shower, a dinner, a Bible study, or even a church service. Although I prayed about it, I honestly could not find true joy at those times without Gary beside me. It was as though the part of me that had become him was absent. Whenever he experienced a more serious medical need, going anywhere, except to his bedside, was out of the question. I thanked God for blessing me with good health so I could be there.

My husband and I bonded in our relationship with one another and, as a three-stranded cord, to God. The cross-stitched wedding gift of our marriage seemed to declare that our precious moments had timeless magic to them. Knowing that life for either one of us could end at any given time, living each moment to the fullest with one another was our main priority in life.

When you pass through the waters, I will be with you; and when
you pass through the rivers, they will not sweep over you . . .
For I am the Lord, your God . . .
Do not be afraid, for I am with you.

Isaiah 43:2, 3, 5

"Christine, let Him have all your worries and cares for He is always thinking about you and watching everything that concerns you."

1 Peter 5:7 (Written in a card from Gary)

Chapter Fifteen

Let Go and Let God

Because teachers rarely get interrupted for a phone call mid-afternoon, I knew that it was UBC Hospital. My heart raced when I heard my name being paged—it could mean anything. The nurse on the other end of the line sounded concerned. "Gary is upset and scared; he needs you here."

"Is he . . . worse?"

"No—he's okay. But he needs to hear your voice. Could you leave right after school?"

There was only an hour of classroom time left but I wanted to leave right then. Going back and trying to teach in a normal mode was next to impossible. My mind was on Gary—he needed me. Once again, I prayed for guidance and strength.

Racing out of school at 3:00 p.m., I arrived at the hospital only to find my husband fast asleep in his hospital bed. "Thank you God," I murmured aloud. It was so good to see him resting. The morphine doses had been on the increase to control the excruciating pain he was experiencing, emanating from his right lung through to his back and abdomen. Originally, the pain was due to a lung infection that was diagnosed in September of 1991 which had leveled off with two new experimental drugs. But the infection had flared up again—even worse. And there was an abscess. What I didn't know then was that a doctor, whom we had rarely seen, had just told Gary, very bluntly, that his lung would never get better.

Despite his high pain threshold, Gary began taking morphine in November of 1991 for the incredibly devastating pain he was experiencing. The side effects of morphine seemed to perpetuate a vicious cycle. Apart from hallucinations, the drug would cause a slowdown of the digestive system, causing the abdomen to be very full which, in turn, aggravated Gary's source of pain. Doctors suggested an intercostal nerve block with a drug called phenol,which, if successful, could block pain in a designated area for up to twenty-eight days.

We agreed to the nerve block and, after an ambulance transfer to St. Paul's Hospital, Gary was under the care of a specialist. This doctor explained the procedure and administered a relaxant to Gary. "We will give him an injection of phenol through his back in order to freeze a local area."

I questioned him, "Is it dangerous?"

"There are risks involved—including the possibility of puncturing the lung, or missing the nerves. And then, again, it simply might not work."

Gary, who was anxious and hurting, decided at the last moment that it might be best if I were not in the room. And so I sat in the waiting room, praying and writing in my journal. I thought how God continually keeps us on our toes, and times things His way. *Had it only been two weeks earlier that Gary and I were trying to coordinate plans for his medical care while I was out of town with my students?* We had been fortunate to make arrangements at UBC Hospital for the week. *Who else, other than the caring staff, could have done Gary's medications twice a day and also been his eyes?*

We had gone out for an early dinner with my family for my birthday, only to be at UBC Hospital's ever-so-familiar emergency ward at 3:30 a.m. There was no choice in the matter—Gary was in excruciating pain. He was admitted earlier than we had anticipated and, although I went to work four hours later, my mind and heart were with my husband. I had not been my happy self—and definitely lacked enthusiasm about going off to Quebec with thirty-three students. My heart longed to stay home; however, Gary, knowing that I could have cancelled, insisted that I make the trip. In retrospect, I think Gary felt that I needed a break from all the medical strain.

I had needed to trust that God would watch over Gary. Knowing that he would be at the hospital instead of home, or staying with someone, had given me a sense of peace. If there were to be any problems, he would be in the right place, with the right people. Gary and I both found the doctors and the nursing staff at UBC to be fabulous and appreciated their support, friendship and care.

I departed for Quebec with two other colleagues and thirty-three students. Speaking to Gary every day that week from my host's home caused my telephone bills to skyrocket. He was in relatively good spirits and, although hearing his voice made me feel better, I shed many tears when thinking of the distance which separated us. How I longed to be with him! Thankfully, there were many people who made a special effort to visit him that week. One of his sisters, knowing I was away, had not only been our house sitter but also spent most of her time with him.

Returning home to Gary had seemed like a déjà vu of a couple of years prior, when I had gone on the outdoor education trip with students. Never had I missed anyone so much. Both of us thanked God that we were together again. Every day mattered. Every second was a joy.

I spent the next day at Gary's bedside, returning to work the following day when I received the phone call—the day that had brought me here to this hospital where the doctors were trying to relieve my husband's pain! Earlier that morning, Gary and I had talked about me taking a leave of absence in May so that we could take a trip together. Of course his distress call from the nurse had changed my thoughts to a different gear. *Tomorrow*, I thought, *I must have a letter delivered to the Board Office requesting an immediate leave of absence.*

Finally the surgery was over—but, sadly, the block didn't seem to help much with the pain, and as soon as possible, we requested that Gary be transferred back to UBC from St. Paul's. After the school board received my letter, they were totally supportive of my request for a leave, giving me the option of returning whenever I wanted.

When contemplating an earlier leave of absence, I had asked one of Gary's best doctors, a very kind, gentle listener, for his advice. "What do you think? Shou . . . should I take a leave of absence now?" In reality, I probably wanted him to tell me that it wasn't necessary.

Instead, he calmly responded, "It wouldn't be a bad idea." Soon, afterwards, the same doctor who had upset Gary so much earlier that day, announced very bluntly. "Face it, Gary's lung will never get better."

When the doctors had left and I was alone, I broke down. *I'm being told that Gary could die at any time! God, help me! What will I do?* Though there was a possibility he might carry on for much longer, I knew I had to be realistic—that I had to be prepared.

They've said it to me in concrete, I thought. *Gary is dying.* This ultimate realization hit me in a strange, overwhelming way. But, it was okay to cry; and cry I did. I had never focused much on dying; however, I was now faced with confronting the truth in regard to Gary's mortality.

What if Gary dies now? What if he doesn't get out of the hospital? I want to focus on hope, love and God's plan but what if this is God's plan? I wept, as my mind continued to search for answers. And so my hospital routine began! Nights were spent on a fold-up cot in Gary's room. I worked on report cards late at night and in the early morning so that I would not miss out on his awake hours. The effects of the morphine were quite apparent and the amount of the dosages increased. Family and friends came to visit, mostly on weekends; we treasured the times we could get out for some fresh air and feel the winter sun on our faces.

It was decided to attempt the nerve block a second time. Gary went to St. Paul's Hospital via ambulance where the doctors used liquid nitrogen in an attempt to freeze the nerves that were causing the intense pain. A small catheter was inserted to freeze the area on which they were to operate. I held my husband's hand throughout the entire procedure. His level of consciousness had been in and out over the past couple of days, undoubtedly due to the ever-increasing morphine doses. The agony and pain that he endured those two nights prior to the surgery were torture that I prayed he would not have to suffer again. Neither one of us got much sleep. I was up countless times to fluff pillows, fetch the urinal, wipe his forehead, and offer encouragement as he cried out for relief. We were both exhausted.

When Gary was in the Surgical Unit, I prayed and talked with God, acknowledging my acceptance of the fact that He could take him home at any time. "I know Lord that, if I have to cross this bridge, You will be at my side. You will carry me; You will guide me, protect me and enfold me with Your love. Reality stares me in the face and pulls me down. I know that if the reality of this disease grips Gary fully—if he dies—I have you, Lord."

Another one of Gary's doctors spoke of his courage. "I

have never seen anyone go through so much pain and yet continue to fight the battle. His love of life surely must be the reason!"

How encouraging this was for me. I knew this love of life revolved around God and His love.

Gary's mother shared with me over a tearful late night telephone call. "Christine, Gary is fighting so hard because he loves you so much. He feels that he has everything to live for."

"How I love that man!" Weeping, I realized that I needed to tell Gary he could let go; but, was I ready?

After the second nerve block, the hours in the day were spent sleeping deeply, punctuated by minutes of alertness where I could ask questions and Gary would eat small amounts. At this point, I was still hopeful, yet beneath my hope stung the reality of "what if." I spent the days and nights at his bedside, managing to snuggle up close in the chair: he in the bed and me leaning against mounds of pillows and the side rail.

One of the doctors confronted me on that first day of March. "In the event that Gary should stop breathing, what would Gary and you want?" The doctor proceeded, in a gentle manner. "Gary is in a final stage, he is hanging on, fighting pain with all his might. However, the underlying problem—the infection in his right lung—is not getting any better; in fact, it is worsening. My goal is to make him as comfortable as possible in the light of the fact that there is still no cure for AIDS."

The doctor left the room, sensitive to my need to absorb the weight of the question.

I spent time crying at Gary's bedside, holding his hand, his arm, and resting my head against his. He slept soundly and, eventually, I did, too. It was not until later that I saw the doctor again and spoke to him. "Gary, knowing that resuscitating him would simply be a vain effort, wouldn't want it done. There would be so much distress. He would want to die naturally and peacefully. When it is time, he will know."

Was I deciding his fate? I struggled with the thought, quickly realizing that God was readying me for Gary's death.

There were so many tender moments. In tears, I told him how much I loved him. "When you get to Heaven, will you watch over me?" I could barely get the words out clearly and, in between sobs, repeated myself.

Gary, at this point, was weak and unable to speak clearly. He stretched out his arms as I moved in closer, put his arms around me, patted me on the back and whispered lovingly, "Yes, of course."

We were still able to laugh. Gary's sensitivity and sense of humor were always with him. Although in a hazy state due to the morphine, his request for croissants and lattés accentuated the preciousness of one of our many happy memories. He had not been responding very much over the last week when I tearfully affirmed how much I loved him, admired him, and had learned from him. He put his arms around me as if to say it was all going to be okay. There were tender kisses, more hugs, tears, and talk. His smile was radiant. Gary was thinking clearly and, as usual, loving deeply. Oh, how I loved him!

That night, as he drifted off to a restful sleep, snoring soundly, part of me thought that God would take him before morning. Gary seemed so at peace—content, and finally comfortable. I believe in miracles, and knew that God could cure Gary at any time; however, I also felt at ease and was prepared to accept that His will might be for him to be taken home. Again, I repeated what I believed he needed to hear. "God wants you Gary. I know you will watch over me and, most of all, that God is always with me and He will continue to guide and strengthen me."

My thoughts returned to the time when I had first met this man who would be my husband and how I had admired him. He was a different kind of man, filled with a zest for life, desiring to taste and enjoy it fully. He loved the simpler things. No one could doubt that he had a very big heart and, in answer to my questions and prayers, he had, over the years, let God enter in. We had learned so much from each other. He taught me to appreciate life in its simplicity—not to worry, but to give my worries to God in total trust. He would take care of us and all would work out for good. A friend's words written in a card sent to Gary and me said, "God is always in control, God is always good and God is always right."

Preparing myself through prayer, I had come to terms with the fact that Gary was probably not going to come home to 18th Avenue and Crown. As these thoughts crept in my mind, the impact that this would have on me seemed to crescendo. *Would I want to put an effort into staying at our house? Would I want to keep it tidy, welcoming, warm, filled with love, a garden of flowers . . . without Gary? Yes, I* thought, *Gary would find joy in me gardening.* In my journal, I wrote, "I'll do it for him, for his love of life, love of color, love of flowers, love of people."

Thoughts of myself, alone, in our house, and in our bed brought to mind other questions. *Would I be lonely? How could I go on without my soul mate?*

Somewhere, from within, God provided reassurance that I would need only to turn to Him and think of His promise and plan for me. He would strengthen me, give me courage and renew the zest for life that Gary and I had always shared.

That night I prayed for God to grant Gary restful sleep that was void of pain—also a sense of peace that would enable him to be with the Lord if this was His will. God had truly enabled me, paving a road for me to follow in faith and giving me the inner strength to "let go" when it was time. I knew He would do—was doing—the same for Gary.

The next day was a very emotional one. It had been exactly one month since he had been admitted to the hospital and he was clearly suffering. He moaned in pain for at least twenty hours, nonstop, seemingly afraid, anxious, in pain and distressed. His breathing was so rapid, every breath a struggle, a fight for life. I knew he was fighting because of his love for life—his love for me. Several times I repeated, "You don't have to fight so hard, Gary. It's all right. You can let go and go to Heaven whenever you are ready. I'll be okay. God will take care of me."

Some of Gary's exhaustion rubbed off on me. Tears were invisible to all those who called on the telephone that day. However, anyone who walked in the room got a tearful, emotional hug. It was so comforting to see people and to know that their thoughts and prayers were with us. So many friends had spent much time with us, with me. I am a very blessed lady. Other people have to go through this alone.

Gary had been straining for his breath all day, hardly a sound came from him, and he did not eat nor drink. When he did try to have a sip of juice, it was extremely difficult for him to swallow. His head was turned toward me; and I had been holding his hand, stroking his arm and forehead all day. Family and friends had come to visit.

God chose me for Gary and him for me. He chose us specifically and especially for one another. Gary, my precious husband, took his last breath on that Saturday afternoon, March 7, 1992. Our life together as a married couple was short but very blessed. Apart from the disease, there is nothing I would change, nothing I regret. When I sensed Gary was in a deeper struggle for air, I buzzed for the nurse.

"Please, quick! Call the nurse, get someone!" I cried, shaken, as I sent the visitors out. I witnessed Gary strain for his last breath, then he was quiet. Silence. Stillness. Only a few seconds. The nurse arrived and, as she pulled out her stethoscope, confirmed what I already knew—Gary had died.

She looked at me sadly. "Yes, he has." As an overwhelming sense of loss struck me—loss of my partner, my lover, my husband, my very best friend ever, I began to cry and cry.

It was important to me that I stay in the room for a time. Such an odd feeling to be with someone at the moment of their passing from this world to the next. I wept as I held him, my tears wetting his face. Crying, I repeated, mostly for my comfort, that he was going to Heaven to be with the Lord. His Heaven was now bigger than his weakened body. My tears of heart-wrenching sadness were also tears of joy. This part of life was something we had talked and wondered about so much in the past. The hope in death is new life. Gary was no longer suffering. I pictured him close to Jesus, to God, as though in a beautiful meadow with many flowers all about. Although I could humanly visualize this scene, I know Heaven's reality is far more beautiful, joyous, and peaceful than anyone could ever imagine. I prayed; I cried; I prayed, thanking God for many things about Gary—for what he had taught me—shown me—and what I would draw upon all of my life.

A friend walked in moments later, asking if I needed to be alone. She waited outside the room. I continued to pray. My legs were weak, giving in. My sister Brigitte arrived soon thereafter. A nurse had called her. We prayed together as I continued to hold Gary's hand. Then we returned to my home. Gary's wedding ring was snug in my pocket; the words, "Dieu nous unit" forever engraved on the inside.

Family and friends spent the evening with me, hugging, crying, laughing, reminiscing and praying. As I lay in bed that first night, I prayed, "God, You continue to direct me, to guide me and to strengthen me in all walks of my life."

Trust in the Lord with all your heart and lean not on your own under-standing; in all your ways acknowledge him, and he will make your paths straight.

Proverbs 3:5-6

"Love is what you've been through with somebody."

Chapter Sixteen

Death is Part of Life

The few days following Gary's death were sun-filled, warm and, although forecasts called for rain, the sunshine colored what could have been very gloomy spirits. My days and nights were punctuated with tears and the harsh reality of Gary's absence from my side; yet, at the same time, I felt the joy of him present with our Lord, our God, free of all earthly suffering.

Family and friends dropped by, offering their time and pouring out their love. We hung paintings together, the last task left since moving day in January. Gary and I had planned where most of his paintings were to go; however, I had been waiting for him so that we could do it together. Daffodils that Gary and I planted in January (yes, rather late, we knew) bloomed March 7.

Despite the beautiful signs, it seemed very odd to me that I was to take charge of the necessary funeral arrangements. *Could I possibly do all that had to be done? Could I think clearly? Accomplish anything?* In the past, things of this nature were always done by somebody else, but this time it was just me—not Gary's parents—not my own parents. Although Gary and I had talked about death and writing out a will in the event that one or both of us should die, nothing was ever put on paper. I recall once, in our most recent home, the two of us sitting together in front of a warm glowing fire, attempting to write out a will. We never made a dent in it, let alone finish it. It simply was not a priority. And, to be truthful, for us to think of a will, made us deal with, not only the possibility of Gary's dying before me but, at that point, the probability. A certainty in the midst of uncertainty.

After some consulting with Gary's parents, I decided what shape the memorial service would take, tapping the knowledge in my heart as to what Gary would have wanted. My dad helped me tremendously by proofreading what I had prepared for the newspapers, accompanying me to the funeral home where decisions of cremation, memorial service, church, cemetery, procedures and costs had to be made. He drove me to the cemetery, and there, with Gary's mother, we went over details involving a plot and what was to go on the plaque. My head was very heavy; I was exhausted.

Sitting on the back deck that warm afternoon, listening to some inspirational music, I began to formulate what I wanted to share with those present at the memorial service. With my emotions tugging at my heartstrings, I cried several times prior to even putting pen to paper. There were pauses in the midst of my writing as I called on God to steady me through this time. Reading my words aloud as a practice was very difficult to do without breaking down, but I knew God would give me the courage and stability that I needed to stand strong.

The morning of the memorial service, I prayed and relaxed on the back deck. Somehow God would see me through this day of remembering Gary. I felt so very much at peace that morning, praying that God would help me get through that day when I would later greet people, hug, and, undoubtedly, share tears.

I was overwhelmed and warmed to the heart by the number of people present at my husband's memorial service. Our small church was bursting at the seams and I felt God's peace settling in. There was the inward assurance that He was with me. Although it was challenging for me, our minister suggested that I be the one to conclude the service. I agreed, knowing that God was my strength and very real help. Peacefully and, in confidence, I walked to the podium.

There were some people who, undoubtedly, must have questioned the wisdom of my participation. *She's going to speak? How could she possibly do it without falling apart?*

What a gathering! With standing room only, between 300 and 400 familiar faces had their eyes focused to the front, waiting on me. My first reaction was a barely audible, "Wow." I had paid no heed to the church filling up behind me. Apparently the lineup along the sidewalk had been a sight as people filed in, stopping to sign the guest book. Speaking from my heart, I felt empowered and encouraged, assured that Gary was pleased with the service and my sharing.

Feeling great warmth and love, I thanked people for being there, and then continued on with this message:

> I want to share with you what has helped Gary and me find strength through our struggles. Gary and I always had, and I always *will* have, God as the Rock of our relationship. We learned to "Let go and Let God" in regard to His will for us, plotting the course of our lives together. These days have been the happiest days of my life. I've been blessed. We always knew that God had a very special plan for us as a married couple, and God has a plan for each one of us as an individual. The awesome thing is that God's plan is far better than one we could ever imagine. I can only agree with what Gary often said: "Put your trust in God, and believe things are going to work out." I know they do. I know that Gary is no longer in pain, no longer fighting for his

life here on earth. Gary is in Heaven with Jesus our
God and Savior, rejoicing. He will always be with me.

Gary, je t'aime. Dieu nous unit. God unites us.

After I returned to my seat, the minister closed with a
final prayer. Then, as music resounded from the front, I left,
feeling very lonely and rather odd, walking down this aisle
unaccompanied, not having Gary physically at my side. The
last time I did this in a church was at our wedding as a bride.
This time, a widow.

It was deeply touching to be with my family, friends, colleagues and students who were gathered with me that day.
Though I hadn't really given it much thought, the opportunity
to speak from my heart and to share my grief and feelings
with all of these people was a blessing. What an incredible
feeling of comfort! The sun shone brightly outside and in my
heart, too. Although the day could have been drab and dreary,
my heart was singing and light, feeling such a bond with Gary,
sharing the reality of his present existence. Through his illness, he had been an inspiration to so many people.

During the following days, weeks, and months my
thoughts would often find me longing to be with Gary. Feelings of being alone in a crowd would envelope me over and
over again. But that was just me thinking—no longer of God's
will. His will be done. I am quick to realize how truly blessed
I have been with a man who loved me so deeply, a man with
such a kind, generous and loving spirit. I would not trade our
marriage, albeit short, for anything different, because God
stood by us. Of course, we often wished for different health
conditions by which our road in married life would have taken
a different route. *Would our marriage have been as beautiful?* So many happy times, so much laughter, love, sincerity,
generosity, kindness, creativity, silliness, a love of life . . .
with Gary, and ultimately in our relationship.

110

Looking around the house and seeing an object could bring me to tears. Every single thing in our home had a history and held a memory of "us." How blessed I was to have experienced the kind of love that Gary and I shared. *Perhaps it was a bit beyond the norm,* I thought, remembering our sexual limitations and how frustrating it was for both of us. However this taught us to cope and to realize that love is much more than a sexual relationship—it is the total giving of oneself to a relationship. Our love was so committed—so strong—so beautiful. Though we don't always comprehend reasons for some of the events in our lives, particularly life-changing events, we must trust that God's plan is a wonderful plan. He blesses us hundredfold daily but all too often we fail to stop and count.

The following are two selections that were shared with me during the memorial service on March 11. The first was a photocopy with a picture of Gary and me laughing together, passed to me just before the service; the second one was shared with the whole congregation.

When I Must Leave You

Our loved ones never really die
They just go
Beyond our earthly sight
Into that land
Where there is no night.

When I must leave you for a little while.
Please do not grieve and shed wild tears
And hug our sorrow to you through the years,
But start out bravely with a gallant smile;

And for my sake and in my name
Live on and do all the things the same.
Feed not on your loneliness on empty days,
But fill each waking hour in useful ways.

111

Reach out your hand in comfort and in cheer
And I in turn will comfort you, and hold you near;
And never, never be afraid to die,
For I am waiting for you in the sky.

Helen Steiner Rice

Letter to his wife
Henry Scott-Holland
Canon of St. Paul's (1847-1918)

Death is nothing at all . . . I have only slipped away into the next room . . . I am I and you are you. . . whatever we were to each other that we are still. Call me by my old familiar name, speak to me in the easy way which you always used. Put no difference into your tone; wear no forced air of solemnity or sorrow. Laugh, as we always laughed at the little jokes we enjoyed together. Pray, smile, think of me, pray for me. Let my name be ever the household word that it always was. Let it be spoken without effect, without the ghost of a shadow on it. Life means all that it ever meant. It is the same as it ever was; there is absolutely unbroken continuity. What is this death but a negligible accident? Why should I be out of mind because I am out of sight? I am but waiting for you, for an interval, somewhere very near, just around the corner. All is well.

For I am convinced that neither death nor life, neither the angels nor demons, neither the present nor the future, nor any powers, neither height nor depth, nor anything else in all creation, will be able to separate us from the love of God that is in Christ Jesus our Lord.

Romans 8:38-39

"I rejoice with God over the creation of you!"

Card discovered in October 1992

Chapter Seventeen

Dance with the Heavens

We searched for joy but knew enough not to look for it in material things. Gary and I knew the joy of being with each other, and we knew God was with us. Trusting God and knowing His promise of everlasting life gave us that joy and continues to do the same for me today. The Monday following Gary's death, my friend and her daughter were walking past our house, and the three-year-old tugged at her mother's thoughts.

"Can we go visit Gary and Christine?"

"We can visit Christine, but Gary is now with God, in Heaven."

Puzzled, but quickly offering a solution worthy of a three-year-old, she queried, "Well, when is he coming back?"

"Because he died, dear, he will not be coming back."

Still not fully satisfied, the child suggested, "Well, can we go to Heaven and visit him?"

A challenging job, motherhood! My friend now had the task of convincing her daughter that you don't rush your time to get to Heaven.

We have other friends who owned a small helium tank. Their two children both enjoyed making helium balloons for birthday parties or for other special occasions at their home. Sometimes, they filled balloons with helium "just because." The youngest daughter, also a three-year-old, accidentally let a balloon float away outside. Gone! *Would this not be the thinking of a three-year-old?* But, it wasn't! Instead, she announced, "That's okay, the balloon will go to Gary in Heaven. All balloons go to Heaven."

A few weeks later, the girl's grandfather passed away, and, this time, complete with notes and name tags, balloons were sent to Gary and Pa who were, undoubtedly, having tea together in Heaven.

My six-year-old niece drew a picture for me the day she was told her Uncle Gary had died and gone to Heaven. Her retelling of the story moved me so; it revealed God's truth and love in the most simple terms. The picture showed Gary lying under the ground, smiling, grass and flowers over top of him clad with happy and sad faces. I was kneeling to the right, and Jesus, underground too, was under where Christine was kneeling. Two angels, a happy one and a sad one, were high in the sky. A portion of my niece's message is as follows: "The grass told you that God loves you . . . They're happy and they talk . . . they're telling you that Gary is in Heaven and he still loves you. The angels, one was sad because Gary died and the one was happy 'cause he told you that everyone loves you. God loves you and then Gary loves you and they love you all in the heart . . . and His (God's) heart is full of love . . . and then he says, 'Oh, I love everyone. God, Gary, Christine.' "

Yes, I have learned, through the eyes of children, the simplicity of the joy of everlasting life. Also, I have learned from them a little bit more about God's promises, and the hope that we have in Jesus Christ.

On my way home, after baby-sitting a niece and nephews for the day, I felt worn out and emotionally drained. I was missing Gary. The radio was broadcasting a children's radio show and, in the past, I had always switched the station; however, for some reason, I left it on, intrigued by the story: A young girl, Donna, and her friend, Mr. Wittaker, were off to visit Karen who was in the hospital with cancer. The two twelve-year-old girls were the best of friends and missed being around one another. Karen spoke of being out of the hospital as soon as her chemotherapy was over, and was excited about the school fair since she would be doing a song and dance. In the meantime, her peers at school assumed that hospital-bound Karen would not be able to make the fair. One day, soon thereafter, Donna learned that Karen's cancer had gotten worse and that her leg had to be amputated.

I thought, *How ironic that Gary, too, was an amputee at a young age.* Now drawn into listening, I wondered if there was a message for me in this story. Donna went to visit Karen again and they talked about how Karen was feeling, school, Karen's cat, and once again, the school fair. Karen was adamant that she would be out of the hospital in time to attend the event. Although, she still wanted a part in it, obviously, the dance routine was out.

When the day of the fair arrived, Karen's cancer was in remission and she was on stage reading a poem. It was a selection that her grandfather had read to her as he rocked her to sleep as a young child. The poem, based on an old hymn, *In the Land of Fadeless Days,* struck me about heaven and hope. It depicted the land of fadless days wherein lies the city, four-square where there are gates of pearl, streets with gold, no death, pain, or fears. God would wipe away the tears in this place where there is no night.

(based on Revelations 21:16 ff)

For the second time, I cried, picturing Gary with every

word she spoke, and wondered if I should pull over just to listen to the rest of the story. I decided to continue driving as I was going to take care of another family's children that evening. They were expecting me at 7:00 p.m. The story continued:

Karen's cancer was soon back, worse than ever. Donna came to visit again, and this time conversation revolved around death. Donna pleaded with Karen not to die, but to continue fighting. After all, what was she going to do without Karen? It was not fair that Karen should die. Donna wanted Karen to stop talking about dying.

Karen had accepted the fact that she was going to die. She was obviously not afraid as she said, "I think the doctors think I'm going to die . . . maybe I will. It's OK . . . you will too one of these days . . . no matter what happens now, we'll see each other again because we both love Jesus. Sooner or later, we'll be in Heaven and then we'll have all of forever to be friends."

All of forever echoed over and over in my mind. For the third time in that short half hour, I was overcome with emotion and flooded with the reassurance that God was trying to tell me something—something I already knew, but something so wonderful to hear through a child at exactly the right time. I pulled into my driveway just as the story ended, ran inside for some kleenex, and headed for my second baby-sitting job of the day.

The house we began renting in January of 1992 had a very neglected garden—in desperate need of some TLC. When Gary was last in hospital, I had questioned him about the garden, hoping to encourage him. "When you come home, what kind of flowers should we plant in our garden beds?"

"Petunias," he answered rather matter-of-factly.

"Petunias? We've never planted petunias in our lives, why would we want petunias?"

There was no response, so I said, "No problem, we'll

plant petunias."

A week after the memorial service, I decided I would scatter some of Gary's ashes in the Pacific Ocean just off the beach. Although I knew that there was no hurry, I felt right about doing this. At peace. And very peculiar things happened that day.

Rather heavy-footed, I strolled along the beach in West Sechelt. Private access to the waterfront produces an immaculate beach which, that day, was penciled with logs warming up to the westward sun. My goal was to make my way gently to the rocky bluff at the tip of the crescent. Remembering previous visits to this place with Gary brought back wonderful memories, but it also intensified my longing to be with him now. Feeling heavyhearted, I headed for the bluff, momentarily distracted by a little plastic plant label which I assumed had washed up on the shore. I recognized it as one of those that contain the picture of a plant, its name, care instructions, and a description. *Just litter,* I thought, walking on by. But then, for some reason, I turned around to take a closer look. The label seemed to be peering out at me, reminding me of the gardening I had done just the previous week.

Bending down, neck craned—low and behold—***petunias***!! I just had to take a few steps back and pick up that tag! Tears of joy and indescribable emotion overcame me as I turned towards the ocean as if to thank the waters, God and Gary for the sign.

Elated with joyous thoughts, I quietly prayed for more signs along my unknown road in life. The tag, now snapped in two and carefully taped in my journal, had definitely been in the ocean for some time. It was weathered, bleached and very brittle. *Had I not gone for a walk on that day, at that time, at that place, would the tag have been back in the ocean?* Coincidence? God incidence.

Despite poor weather predictions on this day at Sechelt,

117

the water was calm with the sun burning ever so warmly through the March haze. It was now time for me to go out in the row boat and scatter the remainder of Gary's ashes. On the rippled glass sea, I saw two seagulls in the distance and, beyond that, one of the three Trail Islands that Gary and I had rowed around in years previous! Peaceful, I felt ready to scatter the ashes in the ocean—an ocean Gary loved to walk along, cycle by, or swim in—a part of the ocean Gary and I loved to come and visit. This scattering was completely symbolic; however, I knew that whenever I was near the ocean, I would think of Gary. This warmed my heart.

Once I scattered the ashes, I felt compelled to write what I had just seen. Rowing back to shore with my eyes fixed on the location where I had scattered the ashes, two seals suddenly appeared. One emerged before the other, then together they began to swim about, slipping through the water, crisscrossing each others' paths in their play. "The same way peoples' lives do," I murmured aloud. "How very symbolic, a Gary seal and a Christine seal."

Although I wasn't searching for symbols that day, I knew this was rather special. I quietly tucked the oars in the boat and decided to watch the seals. One took a plunge, the other idled above water, looking about, and swimming. She was going about her own business. I studied that seal, wondering what would happen next. *Would the other seal reappear for air, or would this seal take a dive, too, joining the partner?* I watched as the latter happened. I, too, will be joining Gary one day with God, but, for now, the Lord has more in store for me here on earth. I know the seals meet up, and I also know that they eventually come up for air. This was the same area where I had scattered the ashes. Coincidence? God incidence? All is well.

"If only. What if." Because these two clauses can imply doubt, fear and even a degree of sadness, I learned to avoid using them, focusing instead on my blessings. Before our

marriage, all the uncertainties of our future crossed, not only our minds, but the minds of those people with whom we shared our situation. When one is painted a dark picture and a bleak future, when the disease one carries is AIDS, one cannot help but think, *What if Christine and Gary don't make it? What if she contracts the disease through some cause that is yet-to-be-discovered? What if he dies?* Dwelling on what could happen or what might have been offers no solution. Encouraged by God's word to dwell on the positive, we depended on Him for everything.

Gary was a gifted pianist. Although he did not like to perform, given a relaxed day at home, he would sit at the piano and play from his heart, seldom using sheet music. One of my fondest memories, perhaps more of a feeling, is Gary seated at the piano in the living room of our house on Collingwood Street. On a summer day the music, wafting through open windows and doors, would infiltrate my inner being and bring joy to my heart. No matter how hard I try, I will never be able to reproduce that tune on the piano. When Gary played the piano, he truly made music in the air, in my heart. Not even a week after his death, I thought, *If only I had taped one of those sessions . . .* Knowing that dwelling on this would not bring me happiness or comfort, I dismissed it from my mind, content that the memory of the *feeling* of his music would live in me forever.

As I was digging for winter gear downstairs, I had one of our favorite Acappella tapes playing on the stereo in the living room. Friends had invited me for my yearly token day of skiing at Whistler Mountain and I was trying to get ready. When the music ended, I ventured upstairs to flip the tape. *Homemade tapes . . . not always a professional job,* I thought, noting that the first side of the tape was not filled. After flipping it, I had to push the rewind button, set it, then go downstairs to tackle my job again. The music ended for a second time and there I was still packing—feeling too lazy to go upstairs to change the tape. It was well past my bedtime; I was all alone, enjoying the quiet peacefulness, twenty minutes of total silence. *Then I heard it.* Faintly at first, then it played crescendo. It was Gary on the piano! Yes, at the tail-end of the second side of this homemade tape was a recording of my husband at the piano. I stood, first dumbfounded, then in awe, at the bottom of the stairs and began to cry. How moved and elated I felt! I could hardly believe my ears. *Another blessing?* Yes, I am a very blessed lady.

Although the musical number on tape is not the one I hear in my heart—the one so reminiscent of those warm summer days—it has perhaps far more impact. The song *Change My Heart Oh God* had always meant a lot to both Gary and me for many years. Today, it moves me to tears. In Gary's music lies its melody.

Change My Heart

Change my heart oh God
Make it ever true
Change my heart oh God
May I be like you

You are the potter
I am the clay
Mold me and make me
This is what I pray

Change my heart oh God
Make it ever true
Change my heart oh God
May I be like you

Eddie Espinosa

© 1982 by Mercy Publishing

I thank God every time I remember you.

Philippians 1:3

120

"May our Lord Jesus Christ Himself and God the Father . . . encourage
your hearts and strengthen you in every good deed and word."

2 Thessalonians 2:16-17

Chapter Eighteen

You Won't Believe It . . .

A place has a way of growing on you. The first time Gary and I went to Sechelt together was Thanksgiving weekend in1987 where we camped out on the porch of a friend's family cabin. The water just below the retaining wall lapped up our conversations. West Sechelt, Sunshine Coast had a very special spot in our hearts and we always felt welcome at my friend's summer place. The Trail Islands across the water, the sound of waves lapping the pebble shore, and the birds searching the tide's treasures all provided a relaxing atmosphere, away from the business of hospitals, doctors and checkups. It didn't matter what the weather was like or what time of the year it was; it was always perfect.

Ten days after my first solo Sechelt trip, I found myself, once again, strolling the beach of West Sechelt. Having been so blessed with all of the wonderful signs from Heaven, I was not expecting a thing, being there just to relax and gather thoughts. My friend and I walked aimlessly along the shore as an interesting rock caught my eye. Stooping over to pick it up, I knew this was another God incidence. Years earlier, Gary had found a small pebble the size of a dollar coin that, if you used your imagination, resembled a heart. At least we thought so. The pebble followed us with every move, from one drawer to the next for safe keeping. This new-found stone was, beyond any doubt, a heart. Fitting snugly in my hand, the groove at the center proved to be a perfect spot for fingers to settle. I tucked the stone into my pocket, deciding to share my discovery with my friend at a later time. My heart was smiling. A comfy rock.

Since then heart rocks seem to smile at me a lot. It doesn't matter whether I'm fishing with my nephew in the Okanagan Valley, observing one beside a rock that looks like a whale in New Denver, or visiting the shores of Sunshine coast. To this day, my niece and nephews find them, too, and save them for Auntie Christine.

Four months after Gary's death, as I was clearing out some things downstairs in preparation for a potential room-mate, I came across my guitar in its case. I decided to lug it upstairs, wipe off the dust, check the strings and attempt to tune it. Tucked away in papers within the case, not only did I come across the guitar music to *Change My Heart Oh God* but another song Gary wrote. After a few days of feeling a bit low (3rd year anniversary would have been two days later), this was truly another uplifting moment.

Destiny

Not long ago,
I found the Lord
and He found me
So weak and empty
He gave His love
unselfishly

122

> I love Him, Jesus
> He is my Saviour
> He is my comfort, too
> He is my destiny
>
> And then my life
> began to change
> My eyes were opened
> to his world
> My life was filled
> with holy love
>
> I love Him, Jesus
> He is my Saviour
> He is my comfort, too
> He is my destiny
>
> Destiny
> My life had no
> Destiny
> But now I see the light,
> The brightest holy light
> Clean, strong and purest light
> The light of my destiny.

Music was seemingly becoming a theme in my discoveries. To shorten the drive between Vancouver and Bothell, Washington, where friends awaited my arrival, I decided to replay the tape Gary had made for our wedding. After listening to Louis Armstrong's classic, *What a Wonderful World,* the last song on the cassette began to play. Though my eyes were blurred, my ears seemed to be supernaturally in tune to the words of *Tout ce que j'aime* which accompanied the music. It was as though I were hearing them for the very first time. Both God and Gary spoke to me through the tape and, in my heart, I knew I was also speaking to them.

Most of my tears were shed three years before Gary's death when the reality of AIDS hit us. We grieved together. Today, I could be very angry that life dealt us, and me, such a blow, but there is no anger, no denial. God prepared and strengthened me through Gary and his love. Both my husband and I lived a unique experience, and God was with us every step of the way. I also know that He won't leave me now.

As I pored through cards, notes and pre-marriage correspondence, I came across a letter from Gary, expressing how he was looking forward to the happiness we will all share after our life on earth. He wrote something similar on Christmas Day of 1990 in my parents' guest book. This message speaks to me even more deeply now:

> Again our parents have provided us with a warm home filled with conversation, delicious food, friendship and love . . . we look forward to that day when we gather all together in the presence of our Heavenly Father. Merry Christmas and a Happy Birthday to Jesus.
>
> Gary and Christine

As Gary and I shared our story, we became like an open book, people aware of a very personal part of our lives, as well as the restrictions imposed on us. Although people could "see" our love for one another, I still treasure our secrets, dreams and special times that no one else ever need know about. As time heals, it becomes easier to share our story with people. "Our story" is evolving into "my story." I am now on my own; however, Gary is still a popular topic of conversation—people continue to show interest in him. There isn't a day that goes by when I do not relate myself to my husband in some way. In bed, during the quietness of night, I wonder in awe what his life after death is like. Upon awakening, I am surrounded by his paintings and all the other possessions we shared; I think about him, miss his warmth and his touch. I miss the physical Gary. With excitement and fascination, I think about where death took him . . . his inconceivable place . . . this state . . . Heaven. Until his death I never reflected much about life after death, about Heaven.

Although I know people who have died, Gary is the closest to me. It feels as though part of me is missing. In my limited, human capacity, I try to visualize Gary, God, Heaven, the beauty, the glory—the list goes on. Euphoria! My mind is so finite, so small, it still wonders . . . In response to all this wonderment and meditation, I, one day, will hear Gary's happy-sounding voice calling me with enthusiasm. "Christine, you just won't believe how wonderful it is. You just can't imagine; just wait till you get here—I can't explain it. You're not going to believe this!"

Because I know that I am still here for a purpose, I pray each day for God's will to be revealed to me a little more. I pray that I come closer to knowing His will for me. *Does being in Heaven mean that you now see the whole picture? God's plan for me?* Gary must now see it and fully comprehend. The best I have ever known of my life is now gone. Over! In the past! What I have to look forward to is my future—God's plan for me here on earth. Knowing that I will see Gary again brings great joy, but that is the future. Christine has to live in the present—in today. It is important to me that I do not lose my commitment to prayer. God wants so much for us to depend on Him in all areas of our lives.

Gary and I prayed a lot over the past few years, there being nowhere else to turn. Now I offer my day to the Lord, because of His wonderful promises. Gary would want me to live each day for what it has to offer—not to live in the past.

How could I wish Gary back? For what? So that he could suffer a little more on earth? Granted, we do not really know what life after death is like, but I do have the assurance that it is far better than the ultimate in earthly happiness. And to think that the one who was my husband is living that right now. Awesome! Gary is living his "eternity" just a bit sooner than some of us.

This brings me to my friend's dream. Gary would often wake me up in the middle of the night to tell me about his fabulous dreams—always something extraordinary. Sometimes, he would let me sleep until morning before sharing them with me. My dreams seldom make any sense to me—most I don't remember.

My friend had a dream on March 7, the night Gary died; however, she didn't learn of his death until two days later. Intrigued, I listened to her retell her dream to me in a telephone conversation several days later. Her quiet, peaceful dream began with Gary and me traveling toward a very bright light. There had been no mention about Gary dying. It was very clear that I was accompanying Gary to ensure that he had the correct address: Heaven.

We reached this tremendous light and were truly in God's presence. Gary was welcomed as a permanent resident; however, God clearly said to me, "Oh, no Christine, you are not to stay now. You must go back, as I have other plans for you."

It was with reluctance that I parted, even though Gary and I knew he was safe, happy, and was fulfilling God's plans. And so I left. Her dream ended there as did our conversation, leaving me in tears.

But there was joy in yet another confirmation that Gary is with God. Our Lord communicates in so many different ways and is ever so present in my life. Life has such temporal limitations here on earth, but it is everlasting after death. Wonderful. Eternal life has already started.

For I know the plans I have for you . . . plans to prosper,
plans to give you hope and a future. Then you will call upon me
and I will listen to you. You will seek me and find me when you seek
me with all your heart.

Jeremiah 29:11-13

EPILOGUE

After finally completing my manuscript I embarked on a seven-week trip to France. I hadn't been back since my trip with Gary in 1989. This time my goal was to visit and spend time with all the relatives I could, particularly with my then eighty-eight year old grandmother with whom three weeks was shared and treasured. It was my wish to touch base with the persons who had questions about Gary's death. I was now feeling strong enough to tell them about AIDS, and how it had affected Gary and me throughout our marriage.

One of my cousins, Marie Odile, was one of the long-distance family members with whom I had maintained a close relationship via mail as well as infrequent visits. I spent a wonderfully relaxing week with her, her husband and their three children at their summer home in La Mayenne, near Brittany, France. Our conversations revolved around life, Heaven, Gary's disease, and death. We dug deep and fast. There seemed to be no barriers, no inhibitors of where our conversations went. The depth of a relationship is magni-fied, I've come to realize, when each person holds faith in their lives. This, we shared openly.

Upon my return home to Vancouver, I was eager to share the most precious thoughts and feelings with those around me, things emphasized in the latter part of my visit with Marie Odile. We had acknowledged that love and relationships are the truly important things in life, and also discussed how one works these out in accordance with the gift of time God allots to us.

I can count on one hand the number of visits I have had with Marie Odile in my lifetime, yet each one was precious, our every conversation was meaningful, and each letter we exchanged seemed to swallow up the time in-between. The friendship was true.

Relationships are not measured in quantity of time, but in the love and care that exists in it, whether it be through phone calls, annual and monthly visits, or daily contact. Life and all its circumstances does not allow us to spend equal amounts of time with all people, but this does not mean we love them any less.

Returning to my new class in the fall, I, and our entire family, reeled in shock to hear that Marie Odile, having been in her young family's new home barely one week and having laid out the children's clothes for the first day of school, never woke up to see that day. *A thirty-three year old mother of three young children.* Over and over I asked myself, *How can this be? What could have happened?* People questioned me, "Was Marie Odile well when you saw her?"

"Yes," I said, "she seemed perfectly healthy; vitality and energy bubbled out of her in the goings-on of a household with three children."

I told myself, *One day, I'll understand—we all will.* I empathized with her husband Thierry, losing a spouse—a tearing of part of the self. But he was both a widower and a father. *How difficult*, I thought, *something that I can't fully understand.* Thierry and I wrote to one another. Then photo albums of summer snapshots made it through the mail in the fall. They recorded precious moments with "maman." A brain aneurysm had claimed her life.

128

I count myself as truly blessed to have been able to live with Marie Odile and her family for a week of their lives. Spending time together berry picking on the trails, and swimming in the local watering hole was wonderful. Though I had gone to France to spend time with my aging Grand-mère— her great-niece who was sixty years her junior, preceded her in death. In hindsight, the blessing of time with Marie Odile is magnified.

I began to wonder if God was preparing me for my own death and shared this thought with a few people. Life had taught me that we ought to be ready to meet our Lord at any time. Having spoken so freely about life and death with Marie Odile, then learning that this special cousin had died; it just didn't make any sense. *Another young person in her thirties! What was God trying to tell me,* I wondered. *What was His plan?*

That fall I carried on with some of my goals, one of them being to undergo an intense training program for a potential "family support" volunteer position at Canuck Place, a free-standing hospice for terminally ill children in Vancouver. I felt I could continue with my four-day teaching work week, especially since my manuscript was complete.

I enjoyed a white Christmas spent in Nelson, British Columbia at my sister Brigitte's new home, where my parents, aunt, and one of my three brothers were also able to be. My only sister, the youngest of five children, had bought a home and settled in the Kootenays, a mountainous outdoor lovers' paradise, set in southeastern British Columbia. Her gentle nature, attentive, thoughtful ways, and listening heart led her to be a well-qualified, and much loved social worker. She was involved primarily with adults with special needs. We were eager to spend this Christmas in her new home together as a family.

Her house, blanketed in snow, was a cozy hearth for us all. The Christmas tree that she topped herself stood tall and majestic with delicate handmade ornaments capturing the glimmers of burning candles. We easily soaked in the love and warmth.

The new year brought a close to our holiday with Brigitte and a renewal to our own homes and jobs. We looked forward to our next family reunion—maybe Easter or spring break. As it turned out, Brigitte was unable to come at Easter. The next-planned trip would be mid-July to help celebrate our father's seventieth birthday at the family cabin near Sechelt on the Sunshine Coast, a drive and a short ferry ride away from Vancouver. Brigitte and I began to make plans to do a cycling and camping trip in the Kootenays after her visit to the coast. We would soon relive some our cycling ventures of France 1985—this time in an area she knew well.

As I looked forward to a summer trip with Brigitte, family and friends were blessed with what I coined "B's Bonus Visit." A conference in Vancouver brought Brigitte to town for several days in June. She shared her time with family, planning overnight stays at various homes, and basking in the love. Together, Brigitte and I did things we didn't often do together: went out for breakfast and dinner, saw a play, and truly enjoyed one another. Although her work-related visit was short, it was surely appreciated. I was touched, upon return from work on the day she left, to find a note of blessing and a gift in my living room. Footprints on my heart.

That note now speaks timeless volumes: "God bless you and your home . . . with flowers of the heart and Heaven: love, peace, joy. Thank you for sharing with me. Simply and freely. I love you. Brigitte." The footprints on my heart have an everlasting impression. Brigitte's eight-hour drive from Nelson to Vancouver was never completed. It was all very quick. The car swerving to the left, a quick correction, back into her own lane, tires screeching, metal smashing metal, crushed, motionless, on the hillside. Car Crash! It was instant and there was one fatality. Someone put a blanket over my sister. She was three hours from Vancouver. Meanwhile our family was awaiting her arrival in Sechelt. A bow was put around the picnic table for our father's birthday. With anticipation, we expected Brigitte to pull into the driveway around midnight. When she didn't, I thought, *She'll catch the first ferry in the morning.*

Then at 4:00 a.m. my distraught brother called; he was the only one unable to be with us on that weekend. Barely awake, I couldn't make out what he was saying. "Eric, is that you? Where are you? Are you okay?" Then I realized it wasn't me being sleepy that was the problem. His speech was inaudible. "Eric. Where are you?" I repeated, feeling anxious and concerned. "Are you with Brigitte? Where are you?"

"Brigitte . . . Bri—"

"Eric, I can't understand you. Are you alright? What's wrong?"

"Police . . . came . . . car accident . . . dead . . ." Then there were deep, heart-wrenching sobs.

As the reality of what he was saying began to sink in, I cried out in shock and disbelief. "No! No!" Numbly, I handed the phone over to my sister-in-law who had heard me crying out. My thoughts were racing, *Brigitte? Not here? Killed? NO!*

One by one, family members made it up the stairs to investigate the commotion. We looked at each other—wanting this to go away, not wanting to accept it. "Are they sure?" someone asked. Then came the wailing from the pit of our stomachs as reality began eating away; we felt raw. Weeping and then a horrible silence. Tears and a devastating feeling of emptiness. *This can't be,* we told ourselves. *Why would this happen? Why Brigitte?* There are so many questions. Search for reason. Empty answers. The only thing we could feel was the pain, the unrelentless pain. We had an open wound; it was so deep.

We spent days talking about Brigitte, trying to make some sense of this reality. Once again, I thought about the gift of time. *It was so precious. Please, God, help me spend it wisely.* With the organizing of the funeral and burial, came the initial acceptance of her death. Then weeks later, we entered and emptied her home of belongings. Each one of us had special memories of Brigitte; we savored them, determined to capture her forever in our minds.

With the distribution of some of her belongings a few months later, there began to be a strengthening of ties in family and friends who see the value of the simplicity of life. *For what do we take with us when we die?* Love! *What did Brigitte leave in abundance?* Also, love! In my finite understanding of Heaven, I know that God is the author of a larger story. Though the pain in my heart and heart-wrenching tears continue, the agony of this separation has lessened somewhat with time and given way to a certain peace in knowing that Brigitte is with the Lord. In fact, I can picture Gary, Marie Odile and Brigitte, wanting to communicate to us how glorious Heaven is. In my thoughts, I hear them, saying, "Carry on with seeking out God's will in your lives." Although I do not understand God's purpose in these deaths, I am given peace, knowing that there is a "big picture" that I will one day understand.

It gives me great joy, as I imagine our loved ones communicating the following words to us, translated from a French poem written by Saint Augustine. It was read at my cousin's funeral in France in 1994, and by me at my sister's funeral in 1995.

Do not weep, if you love me.
If you only knew the gift of God and what Heaven is.
If you could hear, from here,
the song of the Angels and see me among them.
If you could see unfold, before your very eyes,
the horizons and the eternal fields, the new trails where I walk.

If, for just a moment, you could contemplate,
as I do, the beauty which transcends all other beauty.
Well! You saw me, you loved me, in the land of shadows,
and you will not be able to see me again or love me again in the land
of unchanging realities.
Believe me, when death will come to break the chains as she broke
those which imprisoned me,
and when the day that God knows and has set,
your soul will come to Heaven where mine has gone before,
that day—
you will once again see the one who loved you
and loves you still,
you will once again find her heart and all of her tenderness.
Wipe away your tears
and do not weep if you love me.

~~~~~~~

I meet you where our prayers for hope and for Life meet
with the Spirit that sustains us in all trials and joys.

(From a note Brigitte once wrote to me.)

~~~~~~~~~

The hope in death is alive.

July 1996

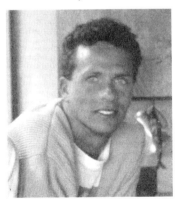

133

ATHLETE PROFILE
GARY SIMPSON

Month/Year	Competition	Location	Event	Standing
08/86	World Aquatic Championships (able-bodied)	Madrid Spain	200M I.M.	Exhibition
08/86	International Games	Gothenberg Sweden	100M Backstroke 200I.M.	World Record World Record
07/86	Canadian Nationals	Brampton Ontario	100M Backstroke 100M Breastroke 200M I.M. 100M Butterfly 100M Freestyle	First Canadian Record First First Second
04/86	BC Masters Championships	Vancouver B.C.	100M Backstroke 100M Breastroke 100M Butterfly 200M I.M. 200M Backstroke	First Canadian Record First First First
09/85	European Invitational	Fulda West Germany	100M Backstroke 100M Butterfly 100M Breastroke	World Record Canadian Record Canadian Record
08/85	Canadian Nationals	Sault Ste Marie Ontario	100M Breastroke 100M Butterfly 100M Backstroke 200M I.M. 200M Freestyle	Canadian Record Canadian Record First Canadian Record First

Named "Most Outstanding Male Athlete" of the Canadian Games for the disabled.

Month/Year	Competition	Location	Event	Standing
04/85	Australian Nationals	Canberra Australia	100M Backstroke 100M Breastroke 100M Freestyle 100M Butterfly	Open Record (1st) Open Record (1st) Open Record (1st) Open Record (1st)
03/85	UBC Special Achievement Award			
02/85	Canada Western University Championships	Calgary Alberta	100M Backstroke 200M Backstroke	World Record (4th) World Record (2nd)
06/84	Olympics for the Disabled	New York New York	100M Backstroke 200M I.M. 4 x 100M Medley	World Record and Canadian Record Third Second
03/84	UBC Special Achievement Award			
10/83	World Swimming Championships	Skovda Sweden	200M Backstroke 800M Freestyle	World Record Second

134

Month/Year	Competition	Location	Event	Standing
03/83	UBC Big Block Letter Award for University Athletes– Only the second disabled athlete to receive such an award. UBC Special Achievement Award			
02/83	Windsor Classic Games	Windsor Ontario	100M Backstroke	World Record
01/83	UBC Tri Meet	Vancouver British Columbia	100M Backstroke 200M Backstroke	World Record World Record
08/82	Pan American Games	Halifax Nova Scotia	100M Backstroke 100M Freestyle 100M Breastroke 100M Butterfly 200M I.M. 400M Freestyle 4 X 100M Medley	First First First First First First First
08/81	Canadian National Games for the Disabled	Scarborough Ontario	100M Backstroke 400M Freestyle 100M Breastroke 100M Butterfly 200M I.M. 400M Freestyle	World Record First Canadian Record Canadian Record First First
06/80	Olympic Games for the Disabled	Arnheim Holland	100M Backstroke 200M I.M. 100M Butterfly	World Record and Canadian Record World Record and Canadian Record Second
08/79	Stoke Mandeville Games	London England	100M Backstroke 400M Freestyle 100M Butterfly 00M Freestyle 200M I.M.	World Record and Canadian Record World Record and Canadian Record Canadian Record Canadian Record Canadian Record
02/79	Canadian Games for the Disabled	St. John's Newfoundland	100M Backstroke 100M Butterfly 100M Freestyle 200M I.M.	World Record Canadian Record Canadian Record Canadian Record
02/78	Named Sport B.C.'s Physically Disabled Athlete of the Year B.C. Sports Hall of Fame			
05/77	Washington Wheelchair Games	Seattle Washington	100M Backstroke 100M Freestyle 100M Breastroke 100M Butterfly 200M I.M. 400M Freestyle 4 X 100M Medley	First First First First First First First
	Chosen "Outstanding Male Athlete of the Games"			
06/77	B.C. Games for the Physically Disabled	Vancouver British Columbia	100M Backstroke 100M Butterfly 100M Freestyle 200M I.M.	World Record World Record World Record World Record
08/77	"Athlete of the Year" by Canadian Wheelchair Sports Association, B.C. Division			

135